ANGIOGRAPHY

Edited by **Burak Pamukçu**

Angiography
http://dx.doi.org/10.5772/intechopen.73817
Edited by Burak Pamukçu

Contributors

Abdel-Razzak Mohammad Saeed Al-Hinnawi, Daniel Emilio Dalledone Siqueira, Ana Terezinha Guillaumon, Behzad Alizadeh, Yakup Balaban, Vincent Dangoisse, Antonio Jesus Guerra, Joaquim Ciurana, Iveta Tasheva, Ivo Petrov, Jivka Stoykova, Liubomir Dosev, Petar Polomski, Burak Pamukçu

Notice

First published in London, United Kingdom, 2019 by IntechOpen
IntechOpen is the global imprint of INTECHOPEN LIMITED, registered in England and Wales, registration number: 11086078, The Shard, 25th floor, 32 London Bridge Street
London, SE19SG – United Kingdom
Printed in Croatia

British Library Cataloguing-in-Publication Data
A catalogue record for this book is available from the British Library

Additional hard and PDF copies can be obtained from orders@intechopen.com

Angiography, Edited by Burak Pamukçu
p. cm.
Print ISBN 978-1-83880-089-5
Online ISBN 978-1-83880-090-1
eBook (PDF) ISBN 978-1-78985-625-5

For EU product safety concerns:
IN TECH d.o.o., Prolaz Marije Krucifikse Kozulić 3, 51000 Rijeka, Croatia,
info@intechopen.com or visit our website at intechopen.com.

Meet the editor

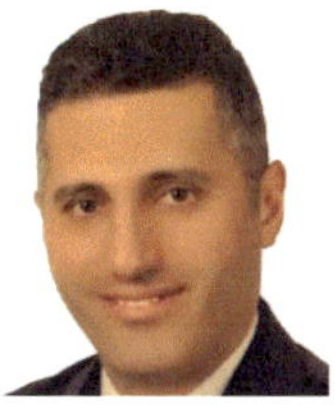

Burak Pamukçu (MD) obtained a doctorate degree in Cardiology from Istanbul University Faculty of Medicine, Istanbul, Turkey. Dr. Pamukcu made his postdoctorate fellowship (European Society of Cardiology Atherothrombosis Research Fellowship) in the University Department of Medicine, Centre for Cardiovascular Sciences, City Hospital, Birmingham, England, UK. He is mainly interested in atherothrombosis, atherosclerotic heart vessel disease, antithrombotic therapy, and interventional cardiology. Currently, Dr. Pamukcu is working as a consultant cardiologist and associate professor of cardiology in Acibadem Mehmet Ali Aydinlar University. He has published 99 scientific publications and served as a referee for more than 30 different medical journals indexed in SCI and SCI expanded. He is serving as associate editor and editorial board member for peer-reviewed medical journals.

Contents

Preface

Conventional angiography is still the gold standard diagnostic procedure for the majority of coronary and peripheral vascular diseases, and therapeutic interventions have advanced dramatically in the last few decades. The evolution of both diagnostic and therapeutic interventional techniques and implementation of new devices (catheters, wires, balloons, stents, valves, etc.) into clinical practice have been important successes in angiography, cardiac catheterization, angioplasty, and modern catheter-based interventions used for the treatment of structural heart disease in recent years. Fifty years after the first angioplasty procedure realized by Dr. Gruentzig, we now have the ability to make successful angioplasty and stenting for left main coronary artery stenosis, bifurcation lesions, chronic total occlusions, and peripheral arterial diseases, including carotid, subclavian, iliac, femoral, and even small extremity vessel lesions. Advancements in the treatment of structural heart and vessel diseases by catheter-based techniques are astonishing and it is possible to close septal defects, to treat aortic aneurysms (EVAR, TEVAR) by devices, or to implant an aortic valve percutaneously (TAVR) with great success.

Coronary angiographic interventions evolved from basic left heart catheterization to complex interventions with the aid of a huge amount of medical industrial material, including differently shaped catheters, guidewires, microcatheters, balloons, stents (bare metal, drug eluting), absorbable biovascular scaffolds, etc. Vascular access sites and techniques have also evolved within the last few decades, and radial access has become the preferred access site for the majority of coronary interventions. Several new techniques are provided for the evaluation of lesion severity, including fractional flow reserve, instantaneous wave-free ratio, intravascular ultrasound, and optical coherence tomography.

In this book we aim to overview developments and innovations in diagnostic, technical, and therapeutic angiographic procedures. Despite all developments in the field, morbidity and mortality from vascular diseases are still very high. On the other hand, we need further advancements for practical treatment of structural heart diseases. Our perspective for the next few decades should be based on preventing vascular disease and providing more successful interventional therapies for patients with vascular and structural diseases.

I hope that this book will support our practical and theoretical knowledge in the field. I would like to acknowledge all contributing authors and our author service manager Ms. Romina Skomersic for their contributions to the project.

Burak Pamukcu, MD
Consultant Cardiologist & Associate Professor of Cardiology
Acibadem Mehmet Ali Aydinlar University
Vocational School of Health Sciences
Department of Emergency and First Aid
Istanbul, Turkey

Section 1

Introduction

Chapter 1

Introductory Chapter: An Overview of Angiographic Vascular Interventions

Burak Pamukçu

Additional information is available at the end of the chapter

http://dx.doi.org/10.5772/intechopen.81768

1. Introduction

Coronary heart disease is the most common cause of death among adults in developed countries, and its prevalence is increasing in developing world [1, 2]. Physical inactivity, obesity, metabolic disturbances including diabetes mellitus, hypercholesterolemia, and hypertension and salty diet, and cigarette smoking are leading to increased vascular diseases [1, 2].

Angiography is still the gold standard diagnostic technique in a majority of vascular diseases. The histories of angiography, cardiac catheterization, angioplasty, and modern catheter-based interventions start in the early eighteenth century. Hales made the first documented biventricular catheterization in a horse in 1711 [3]. Then, Forssmann's right heart self-catheterization in 1929 became a milestone in the history of heart catheterization [3]. After success in right heart catheterization, researchers focused on left heart, and Zimmerman, Cope, Ross, and colleagues achieved left heart catheterization too [3]. The start for coronary angiography was given by Sones in 1958 and was followed and developed by Judkins and Amplatz via femoral access in angiography [3]. In 1963, Dotter accidentally caused recanalization of a peripheral artery with the catheter. In the 1970s, Gruentzig started balloon angioplasty and unlocked the door of vascular interventions era [3]. Several technical and industrial developments allowed us to perform vascular interventions frequently and with great success today.

Current catheter-based interventions are frequently used in cardiology, interventional radiology, and neuroradiology for treatment of aortic, coronary, cerebrovascular, and other peripheral arterial occlusive and nonocclusive diseases. Interventional therapies are also available for a long time in structural heart diseases (e.g., closure of; atrial or ventricular septal defects, patent foramen ovale, or left atrial appendage).

Coronary angiographic interventions evolved from basic left heart catheterization to complex interventions including multivessel, bifurcation, left main, and chronic total occlusion therapies. There is a huge amount of industrial materials including differently shaped catheters, guidewires, balloons, stents (bare metal and drug eluting), absorbable biovascular scaffolds, etc. used in modern catheter laboratories.

On the other hand, the more we understand the coronary physiology, the more we use the evidence-based techniques. For example, fractional flow reserve (FFR) allows us to evaluate the severity of a coronary stenosis (does the stenosis cause ischemia or not) during coronary angiography and guides us whether revascularization is needed [4]. The superiority of FFR-guided revascularization strategy has been shown in recent trials (DEFER, FAME, and FAME 2) over angiography guided strategy [4]. Furthermore, newer techniques not requiring hyperemic stimulation, for example, instantaneous wave free ratio (iFR) can be used today for the evaluation of coronary stenosis [4].

Intracoronary imaging modalities (intravascular ultrasound (IVUS) and optical coherence tomography (OCT)) aim to provide accurate lesion delineation and precise measurements for use during angioplasty. It can provide valuable information while choosing the stent size and best position for implantation [5, 6]. Nowadays, both IVUS and OCT are more frequently used especially during complex coronary interventions (e.g., left main and bifurcation lesions).

Implementation of interventional therapies in daily clinical practice has made the most determinant changes in clinical results of coronary heart disease. Angioplasty and stenting especially in patients with ST-segment elevation myocardial infarction (STEMI) provided important clinical benefits when compared to conventional medical or thrombolytic therapies. At the beginning, angiography was performed via brachial access, then femoral access became the access standard, and now radial access is recommended as the most convenient access site by the current revascularization guidelines [7–9].

In recent years, scientific researches accumulated more evidence to prefer radial access [7, 8] and drug eluting stents (DES) in primary percutaneous interventions [8]. Complex revascularizations during primary percutaneous intervention (PCI) were accepted as contraindicated (class III indication) for a long time, but now, the 2017 European Society of Cardiology (ESC) revascularization guidelines recommend complete revascularization during index primary PCI in STEMI patients in shock with class IIa indication [8]. Another issue, aspiration of blood cloth from the occluded vessel during primary angioplasty (thrombus aspiration) is no more recommended during primary PCI according to the new guidelines. The use of enoxaparin and early hospital discharge are encouraged in patients with STEMI with class IIa indication, while former guidelines were recommending it as class IIb indication [8]. Current advancements in lipid lowering therapy have also affected our practice, and additional lipid lowering therapy is now recommended (class IIa) if low density lipoprotein levels are over 70 mg/dL despite maximum tolerated statin therapy [8].

Current European revascularization guidelines also recommend radial access as standard approach in both angiography and PCI, use of DES instead bare metal stents (BMS) in any PCI, use of Syntax score in revascularization procedures involving left main coronary artery or multivessel disease, use the revascularization strategy preferred among stable coronary artery disease patients in patients with non-STEMI (after stabilization of the patient), use of radial artery grafts over saphenous vein grafts in patients with severe coronary stenosis, and to prefer CABG surgery for patients with coronary artery disease, heart failure, and left ventricular ejection fraction <35% [9].

In this book, we aimed to overview our current diagnostic and therapeutic abilities while using angiography in patients with different vascular diseases. Recent developments in interventional therapies, drugs, and devices provided us great success in the treatment of vascular diseases but we have to learn and progress more. In the future, researchers and developers will keep on fighting against atherosclerotic vascular diseases with the aim of decreasing morbidity and mortality, providing people a healthy life and protecting the well-being of subjects. However, we should not underestimate the value of preventive medicine to achieve more success.

Author details

Burak Pamukçu

Address all correspondence to: bpamukcu@gmail.com

Acibadem Mehmet Ali Aydinlar University, Vocational School of Health Sciences, Istanbul, Turkey

References

[1] Benjamin EJ, Blaha MJ, Chiuve SE, Cushman M, Das SR, Deo R, et al. Heart disease and stroke Statistics-2017 update: A report from the American Heart Association. Circulation. 2017;**135**(10):e146-e603

[2] Global burden of disease (GBD) 2010 study. The Lancet (2012). Available from: http://www.thelancet.com/themed/global-burden-of-disease

[3] Mueller RL, Sanborn TA. The history of interventional cardiology: Cardiac catheterization, angioplasty, and related interventions. American Heart Journal. 1995;**129**(1):146-172

[4] Matsuo H, Kawase Y. FFR and iFR guided percutaneous coronary intervention. Cardiovascular Intervention and Therapeutics. 2016;**31**(3):183-195

[5] Hebsgaard L, Nielsen TM, Tu S, Krusell LR, Maeng M, Veien KT, et al. Co-registration of optical coherence tomography and X-ray angiography in percutaneous coronary intervention. The Does Optical Coherence Tomography Optimize Revascularization (DOCTOR) fusion study. International Journal of Cardiology. 2015;**182**:272-278

[6] Pyxaras SA, Tu S, Barbato E, Barbati G, Di Serafino L, De Vroey F, et al. Quantitative angiography and optical coherence tomography for the functional assessment of nonobstructive coronary stenoses: Comparison with fractional flow reserve. American Heart Journal. 2013;**166**(6):1010-1018.e1

[7] Kiemeneij F, Laarman GJ, de Melker E. Transradial artery coronary angioplasty. American Heart Journal. 1995;**129**(1):1-7

[8] Ibanez B, James S, Agewall S, Antunes MJ, Bucciarelli-Ducci C, Bueno H, et al. ESC guidelines for the management of acute myocardial infarction in patients presenting with ST-segment elevation: The task force for the management of acute myocardial infarction in patients presenting with ST-segment elevation of the European Society of Cardiology (ESC). European Heart Journal. 2017, 2018;**39**:119-177

[9] Neumann FJ, Sousa-Uva M, Ahlsson A, Alfonso F, Banning AP, Benedetto U, et al. 2018 ESC/EACTS guidelines on myocardial revascularization. European Heart Journal. 2018. DOI: 10.1093/eurheartj/ehy394

Section 2

Coronary Angiography and Percutaneous Coronary Interventions

Chapter 2

Minimally Invasive Cardiology for Everyone: Challenging the Transradial Access

Vincent Dangoisse

Additional information is available at the end of the chapter

http://dx.doi.org/10.5772/intechopen.82765

Abstract

Transradial access is now well established as the safest route for percutaneous coronary intervention. Nevertheless, its use is often restricted to "easy" cases, switch to the transfemoral route being too rapidly advocated/mandated. We will discuss the different challenges associated with a "TRA for everybody" strategy. (1) The vascular access per se is challenging. TRA failure is most of the time an operator failure to cannulate this vessel. There are some ways to overcome the technical problems and to improve the operator skill and his success rate. (2) TRA is systematically denied for some patient populations: patients with previous coronary artery bypass graft surgery are particularly at risk of not being catheterized by TRA despite excellent performance of this route for diagnostic or intervention. In the same way, MI patients in unstable condition are also at risk to be catheterized by TFA although, most of the time, their condition is addressable through TRA and will largely benefit from this route. (3) Frailty and small body-sized ill patients are also at risk of TFA for PCI when proximal coronary artery disease must be treated. There are alternatives to the use of large and very large catheters for treatment of proximal coronary artery disease. (4) The radial occlusion is a manageable problem, with simple and effective solutions.

Keywords: transradial access, coronary angiography and percutaneous coronary interventions

1. Introduction

Transradial access (TRA) is now well established as the safest route for percutaneous coronary intervention (PCI) and must be attempted at first whenever possible. In real world, too many cases today are still performed though transfemoral access (TFA). In a case-to-case confrontation, "believers" in the radial way [1] would easily refute common arguments still actually developed by TFA proponents to skip the TRA attempt (or to dash the attempt off): planned intervention better managed/proceeded through femoral access (angiography for a patient with previous coronary artery bypass graft (CABG) surgery being a frequent one), planned interventions requiring large materials/catheters, anticipated lack of support during intervention (a true but often hidden fear for several operators), poor/small/not palpable radial artery, previous attempt failure(s), lack of time ("urgency"), "fast" intervention required for a frailty patient, negative Allen test (it is the most hilarious reason for a radial believer), and finally a failed but often too short attempt.

What is the truth in the background of this resistance? The truth is TRA is not and will never be an easy way to perform cardiac catheterization, the learning curve is long (and never ends), and TRA requires from the operator a true personal investment. Hopefully—and it has to be written somewhere—the return on investments in the TRA technique is large, and succeeding in a difficult case is usually even more gratifying for the physician and his patient when the procedure involved only TRA.

"TRA for everybody" is a personal crusade, and it lets the author to succeed a "non-femoral" vascular route for 1019 of his last 1023 procedures (from mid-March 2017 to mid-November 2018). The 1023 procedures included primary PCI for 152 ST elevation myocardial infarct (STEMI) patients—femoral access for 2 of them—coronary angiography (and ad hoc PCI when requested) for 108 post-CABG patients, and a total of 568 PCI were performed (73% with 5 Fr guide catheters).

Common challenges associated with a "TRA for everybody" strategy and possible solutions must be considered. Subjects being discussed will be:

1. The vascular access.
2. Some patient populations "at risk" to be catheterized by TFA:
    - The CABG population.
    - Myocardial infarct (MI) patients in unstable condition.
    - Frailty and small body-sized ill patients.
3. The radial artery occlusion problem.

2. Access to the radial artery: the vascular access

Cannulation failure, which is the main cause of TRA failure, is disgracefully received by the majority of interventional cardiologists and stays subsequently hidden. And yet it is not a shame to fail the radial artery cannulation: it is a difficult task and so for many reasons. First, the artery is usually small-sized, its diameter being around 2–3 mm [2] depending of the individual body height as demonstrated in one recent study [3]. The arterial wall may be difficult to go through; the vessel may flee away the tip of the needle or may simply "disappear" when a so frequently—and wrongly—invoked "spasm" occurs after a first unsuccessful stick (see discussion below). Although permeable and functional, a radial artery may be unpalpable due to a thick arterial wall or a low flow state. As any other arterial bed, the radial artery is not spared by the inverse remodeling process associated with diabetes, arteritis, and aging. Finally, the patient may be hypotensive with a more difficult vascular access.

So, the first step to optimize the TRA success rate and therefore "TRA for everybody" is investing in solving the problem of the puncture/cannulation of the radial artery.

Data clarifying the causes of TRA failure will now be presented, and secondly, some clues helping in the problem's resolution will be explored.

3. TRA failure's causes

A prospective study about the TRA, conducted by two TRA "believers" and with two major objectives in mind, started in 2015 [4]: firstly, defining the rate of conversion to transfemoral access when the operator must first attempt (and fail) both radial arteries before converting to transfemoral and secondly, the study was designed to record daily and on a case-by-case basis the causes/location of radial artery attempt failure and to define their relative occurrences. The protocol also required grading (1) the ease for cannulation (before catheterization, as assessed at the bedside), (2) the real ease for the attempt, and (3) the ease for the catheterization itself (catheter manipulation).

By protocol, every single consecutive left heart cardiac catheterization, diagnostic or interventional, elective or urgent, has to be first attempted by TRA (right or left or both). Only non-palpable radial artery (on both sides) or abnormal Allen test (Barbeau type D on both sides) and patient refusal were excluded. Let us say immediately that the two operators never encountered a patient with a Barbeau type D present on both sides and that non-palpable radial artery may be permeable and functional as easily assessed with a Doppler probe. Thus, basically, no patient was excluded from the study for such reasons: "TRA for everybody" is feasible at the level of the initial assessment for an arterial access.

As designed by the protocol, all sorts of patient populations were attempted by radial artery, including post-CABG surgery patients, even patients grafted with both left and right internal mammary artery. Some local surgeons also used the gastroepiploïc artery as graft (and not as free graft). Such patients were also included.

Even shock patients were included in the study.

From January 2005 to June 2007, both operators successively and prospectively proceeded to catheterize 1826 patients, starting from right or left TRA, at the operator discretion. PCI accounted for 40% of the procedures. The study was published as an original contribution in the Journal of Invasive Cardiology in September 2010 [4].

The first and major contribution of the study was to offer strong data for the cornerstone of an effective politic of "TRA for everybody": to have to attempt both radial arteries before converting to a femoral access. The study succeeded in offering a "TRA only" procedure for 98.8% of the study population (**Figure 1**). This high success rate was obtained after attempting the second radial artery for the 6.2% missed first radial artery, 4.4% when excluding the patients with previous CABG surgery. Attempting the second radial artery was successful in about 80% of the cases.

As illustrated in **Figure 1**, the study did not identify a special population who will not benefit from TRA. It also dismisses some apprehensions regarding TRA: rate of truly difficult cannulation was half less than anticipated, and difficult catheterizations were 50% less frequent than anticipated (and this rate stays stable at 6%), **Figure 2**.

Multivariate analysis (GEE, RMGEE program, K.Y. Liang and S.I. Zeger, Longitudinal data analysis using generalized linear models, Biometrika 73, 1986) strongly proved the learning curve existence and identified some of the major factors playing in the TRA world, namely, the artery size and a diffusely diseased arterial bed (peripheral artery disease). Four predictive variables for a first radial attempt failure emerged in the study:

- Year of the procedure, variable related to the learning curve, and operators getting better and better with time, OR 0.6, 95% C.I. 0.4–0.8, $p < 0.001$.
- Presence of peripheral artery disease, OR 1.8, 95% CI 1.1–2.8, p 0.016.
- Pre-procedure clinical evaluation for a difficult access, OR 2.5, 95% C.I. 1.3–4.9, p 0.006.
- Small radial artery size as assessed clinically before catheterization, OR 2.6, 95% C.I. 1.4–5.0, p 0.003.

The second major contribution was to reveal that the main cause of TRA failure was not at all related to difficult anatomies as commonly reported and taught (**Figure 3**). At the start of a TRA business, the radial artery cannulation is accounting for about 75% as the main cause to fail. It accounts for 90% of attempt failures when operator had gained more experience. There are several ways to fail an artery cannulation, reflecting the three steps involved: (1) the puncture itself, (2) wiring the needle or the plastic cannula when they sit in the lumen vessel, and (3) after needle/cannula removal, pushing the sheath over the wire.

When analyzing the three different steps, the far most prevalent problem arises at the wiring step: operator reaches the lumen artery, usually with a good blood's backflow, but he cannot forward the wire. Identifying this problem lets to develop better strategies and material (see below).

Thereafter 2007, enrollment in the study protocol was extended, allowing the creation of a large radial access database. With time and experience, more expertise arose [5], and looking at the same data in 2010, failures related to anatomical consideration were actually avoided: failure to cannulate the artery emerged as the cause for 92% of failed attempts (again mainly because of the wiring problem). Crossover to femoral access declined to 0.9% (2010) and is now 0.4% (2017–2018).

http://dx.doi.org/10.5772/intechopen.82765

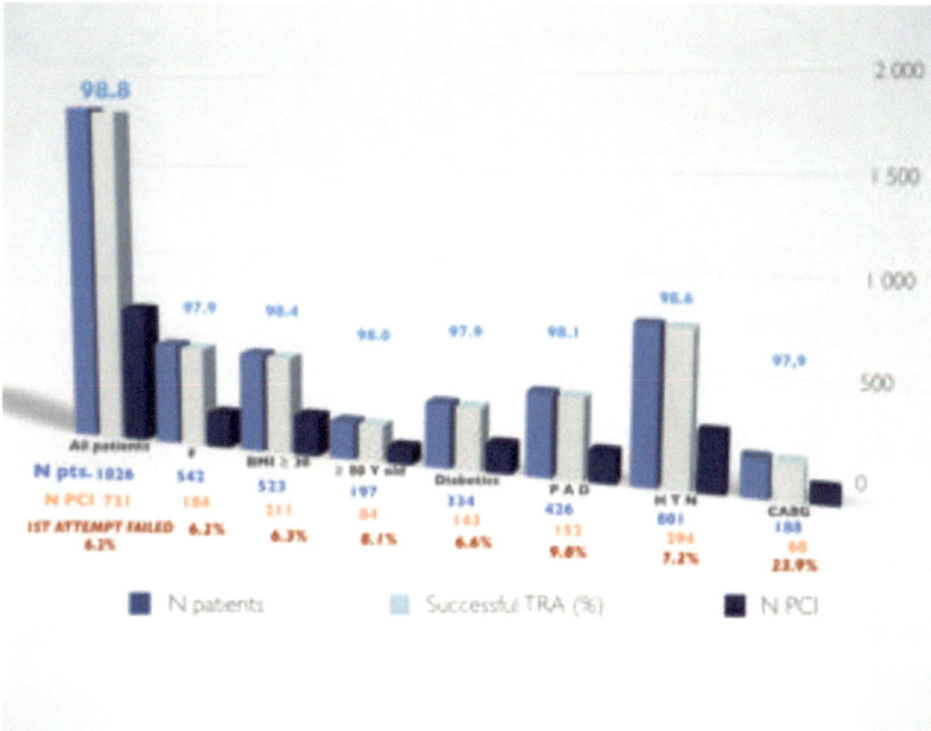

Figure 1. TRA success rate for 1826 consecutive procedures.

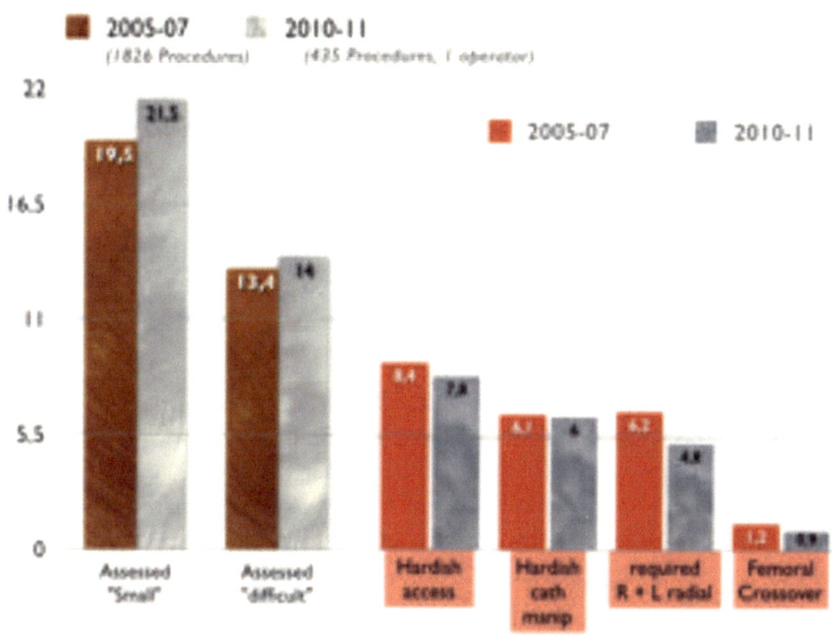

Figure 2. TRA: Real versus anticipated difficulties.

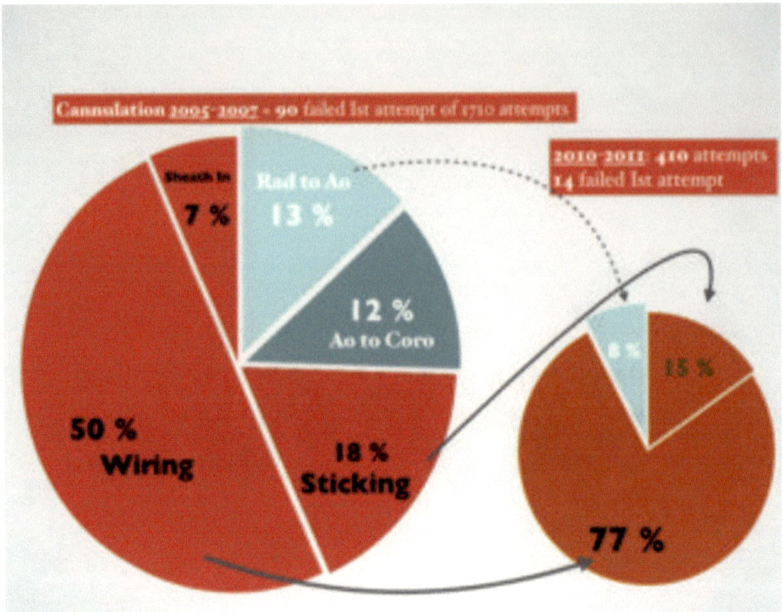

Figure 3. Causes of TRA failure at first attempt.

4. What are the proposed solutions for improving the success rate of radial artery cannulation?

4.1. Utilizing the best techniques and materials for puncturing

Let us talk about sticking the artery, first. Two techniques for radial artery cannulation are at works in the cardiac catheterization world and both gets around 50% of the actual "market."

The first one is derived from the femoral world and is the Seldinger technique. It uses a bore metal needle (usually a 21 Gauge) wired with a short metallic 0.021″ straight or J wire. Its advantage is a sharper bevel, more able to penetrate a stiff arterial wall and a better echogenicity when puncturing with ultrasound guidance. Using the needle with a small body length is recommended: backflow at the hub, signing the puncture success, will happen quicker with a short needle like the Cook® needle 3.5 cm 21 G.

There is a major drawback with the bore metal needle technique: when the standard wire does not progress (either at the needle's entry in the vessel or further away within the artery), the choice for an alternative wire is limited, and particularly all kind of hydrophilic or angioplasty wires may not be used (possible "peeling" of the coating). When you know that more than 75% of artery cannulation is missed because of the wiring problem, it is annoying to lose this possibility.

The second method is derived from the nursing world: it uses an over-the-needle cannula system (needles designed for puncturing veins and intravenous cannula insertion). Insertion of the small cannula within the first mm of the radial artery greatly facilitates the radial wiring and subsequent sheath insertion. Exchange for any hydrophilic or coronary dedicated angioplasty wires is possible and may help and saves many attempts failing with standard wires. The technique is in the author's mind more successful addressing radial arteries of small diameter. Using a 22 gauge system, the vessel injury at the tip of the needle is minimal and allows a through-and-through puncture. The technique is easy to standardize and thus to teach: beginners are instructed to push more deeply the over-the-needle cannula system once the needle reaches the artery lumen (backflow at the hub): doing so, the bevel of the needle is now lying beyond the arterial's posterior wall. Keeping firmly the cannula in place, the metallic part of the system is removed. Then the plastic cannula is gently and mm per mm withdrawn until the blood flows again: the cannula is now perfectly lying in the arterial lumen, and wiring is easier (with the standard or optional wires). For wiring attempts, it is easier to secure in position a plastic cannula than a bore metallic needle. The drawback of the technique is quite minimal: the bevel of the needle is usually not well sharpened for crossing an arterial wall (stiffer and thicker than a venous one); the echogenicity is less than the bore metallic needle (smaller size); some plastics are not well supportive for the standard metallic wire when it has to enter the arterial lumen (all brands of intravenous cannula are not equivalent for that purpose).

Investing in the over-the-needle cannula system, a needle dedicated for the radial access was designed, several prototypes were successfully tested, and the needle is now patented in the USA and Japan and patent pending in the EU [6, 7]. The invention lies in a small distal aperture near the metallic needle tip combined with at least one reinforcing shoulder at the inner surface of the overlying plastic cannula: the system allows a very fast visualization of the tip needle entering the vessel lumen, faster than when you have to wait until the blood flow reaches the more distant needle hub: with the invention, the operator sees first the blood entering the needle's body and then reaching the hub. This feature helps for the first step of sticking the vessel, shortens the cannulation time, and enhances the success rate (no need to re-puncture, less chance to have "spasm" after a first unsuccessful stick). The needle is waiting investors/manufacturers to get in production.

So, the first recommendation for resolution of the cannulation problem is to invest in the over-the-needle cannula technique for puncturing, giving attention to the choice of the puncture material and to the alternative wires.

4.2. Ultrasound-guided puncture

The radial artery is a quite superficial structure easily assessed by ultrasound. The technique requires only a small-sized probe, and setup is easy and fast: puncturing while viewing the artery is obviously easier, and in the most recent author's practice, its use allowed to succeed when blinded attempt had failed. Since its introduction in January 2018 as a bailout technique, and for 439 consecutive procedures, the ultrasound-guided puncture accounted for 43 patients. The visualization of an artery just attempted blindly offered the explanation for the probably most frequent mechanism in play when reattempting unsuccessfully to re-puncture or rewire the vessel: hematoma arising around and within the wall of the vessel, reducing further its lumen (and the pulse). So the "spasm" frequently invoked is in reality hematoma compression/expansion: it explains why the artery is no more palpable and more difficult to re-stick. Furthermore, the ultrasound guidance lets the operator decides to stick at another position or to skip to the ulnar or the contralateral radial/ulnar artery. The ultrasound-guided puncture allows the operator to stick more successfully the artery, but it does not resolve the problem of wiring.

Since many years, as soon as a Doppler signaled the presence of an arterial flow, cannulation of unpalpable radial arteries was attempted. With the ultrasound guidance, it is now far easier to perform this task (and to confirm that the operator may attempt the cannulation, the views allowing the diagnosis of an occluded artery). With the help of ultrasound, the operator may also decide to attempt a less disease or a larger vessel (ulnar or contralateral).

Clearly, the use of ultrasound-guided puncture has a major role to play in a modern strategy of "transradial (or transulnar) access for everybody," and it is the second recommendation for solving the cannulation problem.

4.3. Utilizing all individual resources of the nursing/technologist permanent cath lab staff

You may be an excellent PCI operator and be quite "ordinary" regarding the puncture task (and some hate this fundamental step). On another hand, in every catheterization laboratory, there are individuals very efficient for sticking vessels, and there are individuals well trained for surface ultrasound. A few years ago, nurses interested in the cannulation task were trained for radial artery puncture. The over-the-needle cannula technique was taught, nurses being well customized with this kind of needle and technique. The fundamental difference between their usual way of working with an over-the-needle cannula and for intravenous cannulation is that they absolutely need to go through and through the vessel for a successful radial artery cannulation. They also have to learn the use of the different wires at (good) works. Recently, the same teaching program was successfully offered to technicians in radiology working in the catheterization laboratory: it provided the advantage of adding peoples trained for ultrasound techniques. Actually, the trained nurses and technologists perform 70% of the author's artery cannulations without any undesired crossover to a femoral access.

So, the next recommendation is to train willing and well-skilled nurses and technologists to perform the cannulation task.

4.4. Using forearm artery alternatives (the ulnar artery or the left distal radial artery)

The ulnar artery has been shown to be a safe alternative route for left heart catheterization [8]. It is anyway a safer route than the femoral access and is sometimes larger than the radial artery. It seats deeper and a sensitive nerve is present along the vessel at the puncture level. Hemostasis is easily performed with the material dedicated for the radial artery compression. So, when a radial attempt fails, the ulnar artery cannulation may be a good alternative even at the same wrist. Of course, ultrasound-guided puncture is also an excellent way to optimize the success cannulation rate. Left distal radial TRA is actually in evaluation as a possible way to further improve operator and mainly patient comfort and safety, at least when starting from the left hand. Large series looking at the ease and effectiveness of the hemostasis together with vessel patency and avoidance of ischemic/sensitive problems are mandatory.

The last recommendation will be to become familiar with ulnar artery cannulation, and ultrasound-guided puncture should be a must.

5. Some patient populations "at risk" to be catheterized by TFA

5.1. The population with previous CABG surgery

Patients with previous CABG surgery are difficult to angiography by comparison with non-CABG surgery patients. They are older and have advanced coronary artery disease for many years. Peripheral artery disease and other comorbid conditions such as some degree of chronic kidney failure and chronic obstructive pulmonary disease are frequently found. Graft assessment is an additional task after coronary angiogram and may be tricky due to nonstandard vein graft's ostial location and unavailable dedicated efficient pre-shaped catheters. Arterial grafts are also uneasy to reach: both mammary arteries are originating at a sharp angle from their subclavicular arteries that are to be engaged: the right subclavicular artery may particularly be tricky to reach, except when starting from the right upper extremity. Finally, the gastroepiploic artery, a branch of the coeliac trunk artery, used by some surgeons to graft the right posterior descending artery, may also be difficult to adequately angiography. The additional task of graft angiography and the higher-risk profile of these patients let to more catheters use, more manipulations, and therefore a greater risk of neurological complications [9].

Due to the anticipated complexity of this procedure and concerns about possible greater X ray exposition, TRA—and its associated clinical benefits—is often denied to this population.

Louvard et al. [10] and Yabe et al. [11] reported in 1998 the feasibility of graft angiography and particularly left internal mammary artery (LIMA) angiography through a right radial artery approach. Kim [12] and Kwang [13] described bilateral selective internal mammary artery angiography via the right radial approach as early as 2001. Sanmartin et al. published in 2006 their feasibility analysis and comparison with transfemoral approach [14]. They concluded that there is no excessive delay or greater radiation exposure and that the TRA appears at least as safe as TFA. Their study was retrospective, excluded patients with bilateral mammary grafted, and the left radial access was predominant (133 of the 151 TRA compared to the 154 TFA). They reported four failures of cannulation, one puncture failure, one LIMA, and one saphenous vein graft (SVG) not reached. Only 15% of ad hoc PCI were carried out. In 2008, Burzotta [15] and experienced TRA operators described tips and tricks available for addressing post-CABG patients and already pointed out the right radial access as the best first option in case of bilateral mammary artery grafts.

In 2009, Rathore et al. [16] reported a similar technical TRA success rate for SVG-PCI compared to TFA. Periprocedural MI, access-site bleeding-related complications, and large hematomas were higher in the TFA group. They reported a 5.8% crossover to the femoral route.

The Transradial Committee of the SCAI in a 2011 publication concluded that TRA for CABG patients might safely be integrated into routine practice as experience increases [17].

The published 2010 prospective study of 1826 consecutive procedures [4] looking at the conversion rate from TRA to TFA when both radial arteries have to be attempted before the crossover to femoral included 187 patients with previous CABG surgery. The study was extended for the CABG population until 2012, and results were presented at the 2012 ACC meeting [18].

The study differs from the previously reported series: it prospectively addressed patients with previous CABG surgery; the choice of the radial artery to be attempted at first, right versus left, was free, but both radial arteries had to be attempted before converting to femoral access. Patients grafted with both mammary arteries were not excluded, and the study also included patients with gastroepiploïc arteries used as graft. Ad hoc and elective PCI were performed. Importantly, all causes of failed attempts were analyzed and classified.

This study reinforces the previous conclusions about TRA feasibility. When considering angiography for the CABG population, particularly when only one mammary artery is grafted, TRA performs as well as for the general population. A success rate above 98% was obtained with a very low requirement for a second artery access (7.2%) in case of only one internal mammary artery (IMA) grafted. Of course, the radial artery to be attempted at first must be ipsilateral to the utilized IMA, and it is better to start with in hand the description of the performed surgery. In case of bilateral IMA, the strategy of attempting the right radial artery at first enhances the chance of completing the procedure through one arterial access (actual chance of success is around 60%). To be noted, in the published series, about 35.5% of procedures included angioplasty and stenting (mainly ad hoc). **Tables 1–3** describe the CABG population (from 2007 to 2012) compared to the non-CABG population of the 2010 publication.

To summarize the published statistics, for a general population and excluding patients with previous CABG surgery, cannulation failed in 4.9% (requiring crossover to the second radial artery or to an ulnar artery). For the CABG population when the surgeon protocol is available and when only one IMA is grafted, the ipsilateral to the IMA radial cannulation fails for 5.4% of patients and requires use of the ipsilateral ulnar artery. When both IMA are grafted, starting from the right TRA succeeds for about 60% of patients; 40% will further need cannulation of the left TRA (mainly for an adequate LIMA graft patency assessment). In terms of patient safety and avoidance of vascular access-related complications and hemorrhage, a bilateral radial cannulation is far less dangerous than one femoral access, particularly in case of coronary/graft angioplasty. By the way and as reported [19], the PCI success rate stays unaltered by the vascular access.

5.2. MI patients in unstable condition

The TRA lifesaving benefit is directly linked to the illness severity: the STEMI and the unstable non-ST elevation myocardial infarct (NSTEMI) patients are the more likely to require a high level of several anticoagulants/antiplatelet therapies paving the road for serious hemorrhagic events mainly at the vascular (femoral) access site [20]. Vascular closure devices have not been demonstrated to be effective in reducing these vascular complications in the setting of ACS. On the contrary, hemostasis is easily obtained after TRA, even in situation of

Population	Any previous CABG surgery	Previous CABG surgery	p	Previous CABG surgery ≤1 IMA	p (vs. no previous CABGs)	Previous CABG surgery 2 IMA	p (vs. no previous CABGs)
N	1639	507		320		187	
Age	65 ± 11	71 ± 9	<0.001	72 ± 10	<0.001	70 ± 9	<0.001
Female (%)	31%	18%	<0.001	20%	<0.001	14%	<0.001
Diabetes (%)	17%	29%	<0.001	28%	<0.001	32%	<0.001
HTN (%)	44%	56%	<0.001	54%	0.001	58%	<0.001
Peripheral vascular disease (%)	21%	41%	<0.001	43%	<0.001	38%	<0.001
Weight (kg)	79.0 ± 16	81.6 ± 15	0.001	80.8 ± 15	0.037	83.0 ± 16	0.001
Height (cm)	168 ± 9	169 ± 8	0.26	168 ± 9	0.82	170 ± 8	0.021
BMI	27.8 ± 5	28.6 ± 9	0.001	28.6 ± 6	0.009	28.6 ± 5	0.017
BMI ≤ 22 (%)	10.5%	4.3%	<0.001	4.1%	<0.001	4.8%	0.014
Radial artery looks not easy to puncture	13.9%	12.6%	0.46	13.8%	0.94	10.7%	0.224
Volume of contrast (ml)	156 ± 78	226 ± 92	<0.001	218 ± 87	<0.0001	239 ± 97	<0.0001
Percutaneous coronary Intervention (ad hoc + elective)	40.5%	35.5%	0.04	41%	0.8	26%	<0.001

CABG, coronary artery bypass graft; **IMA**, internal mammary artery.

Table 1. TRA and CABG vs. non-CABG populations.

high anticoagulation level. Performing through a radial artery access in these circumstances removes the fear of "collateral damages" related to intense anti-clot treatments and allows retaining the benefits linked to their use. When the situation requires the use of intra-aortic counterpulsation, the TRA PCI saves at least this access from hemorrhage, the intra-aortic balloon being usually removed some days later, when the degree of anticoagulation is far less intense. Door-to-balloon time is only one of the important lifesaving parameters and must not serve as a pretext to skip a well-performed TRA attempt: speed may not lead to haste! Acute MI patients usually maintain initially a decent radial pulse, and cannulation may succeed as in stable condition. Particularly in the setting of acute coronary syndrome (ACS), a failed first attempt must lead to attempting the second radial artery (or the ulnar artery) before crossing over to the less safe femoral route. The author's most recent statistics in STEMI patients will illustrate the TRA feasibility "in real world."

Since mid-March 2017 to mid-November 2018, from a total of 1023 procedures, 152 STEMI patients were primarily addressed by PCI. A grand total of two primary PCI were performed through a femoral access: one MI patient had previously a thoracic vascular repair after a

	All	Non-CABG patients	CABG patients	p	CABG ≤1 IMA	p	CABG 2 IMA	p	TRA-IMA same side	p
N Patients	2146	1639	507		320		187		298	
TRA success	2118	1621	497		314		183		293	
(%)	98.7	98.9	98	0.13	98.1	0.247	97.9	0.216	98.3	0.395
N radial attempted	2327	1711	616		339		277		311	
N of radial attempts/patient	1.084	1.044	1.215	<0.001	1.059	0.23	1.481	<0.001	1.047	0.981
Right radial as first attempt	1560	1359	201		62		139		41	
Right radial failed at first attempt	139 (8.9%)	68 (5.0%)	71 (35.3%)	<0.001	10 (16.1%)	<0.001	61 (43.9%)	<0.001	4(9.7%)	0.175
Left radial as first attempt	586	280	306		258		48		257	
Left radial failed at first attempt	56 (9.6%)	12 (4.3%)	44 (14.4%)	<0.001	13(5.0%)	0.678	31 (64.6%)	<0.001	12 (4.7%)	0.83
All failures (first attempt)	195	80	115		23		92		16	
One (first) failure/patient	9.1%	4.9%	22.7%	<0.001	7.2%	0.091	49.2%	<0.001	5.4%	0.721

CABG, coronary artery bypass graft; **IMA**, internal mammary artery; **TRA**, transradial access; **TRA-IMA same side**, transradial access for ipsilateral IMA.

Table 2. Radial artery cannulation: failures at first attempt.

	Non-CABG patients	CABG patients	p	CABG patient ≤1 IMA	p (vs. no CABG)	CABG patient 2 IMA	p (vs. no CABG)
N	1639	507		320		187	
N R ± L radial failed (% patients)	90 (5.5%)	119 (23.5%)	<0.001	25 (7.8%)	0.106	94 (50.3%)	<0.001
N puncture/wiring failed (% total failures)	67 (74.4%)	14 (11.8%)	<0.001	12 (48%)	0.012	2 (2.1%)	<0.001
N "route to aorta" failed (% total failures)	12 (13.3%)	5 (4.2%)	0.017	2 (8%)	0.471	3 (3.2%)	0.012
N "coronary or SVG ostium" failed (% total failures)	11 (12.2%)	12 (10.0)	0.625	5 (20%)	0.32	7 (7.5%)	0.276
N "IMA contra not reached" (% total failures)	0 (0%)	88 (74.0%)	<0.001	6 (24%)	<0.001	82 (87.2%)	<0.001

CABG, coronary artery bypass graft; **IMA**, internal mammary artery.

Causes of radial attempt failure, puncture/wiring the radial artery; catheter, route to aorta failure; catheter, coronary/saphenous vein graft (SVG) ostia cannulation; catheter, contralateral IMA not cannulated (right TRA for left IMA or left TRA for right IMA).

Table 3. TRA CABG vs. non-CABG, causes of failed attempt.

thoracic trauma (car accident): his right arm was unavailable for left heart catheterization, and cannulation of the left radial artery led to an occluded left subclavicular artery. The second femoral case was a small-sized lady, and the attempts to wire radial (and ulnar) arteries failed at both wrists. This case happened before the availability of the ultrasound technique for rescuing the failed attempts. Seven STEMI cases required simultaneous use of the femoral artery for left ventricular assistance (intra-aortic balloon pump). The hemorrhage-saving TRA feature lets to more liberal use of potent antiplatelet drugs and high heparin doses: it may lead to less distal thrombus embolism and less no-reflow post-reperfusion states. As already stated, femoral access accounted for only 4 cases of the last 1023 author's procedures.

5.3. Frailty and small body-sized ill patients

There is another category of patients likely to get catheterized by the femoral route: the small body-sized ill patients, particularly if a frailty condition is associated. Excuses to skip the radial access stay similar: anticipated—but not objectively assessed by ultrasound—too small radial artery, need of a large guide catheter for a quicker intervention, speed required by the degree of illness, etc. Nevertheless, this kind of patient will very badly recover from any hemorrhagic event, and their condition increases greatly the vascular risk [20]. The reader is invited to look at the way a cohort of such frailty; old and severely diseased patients were successfully TRA managed through a double radial route for addressing distal left main or proximal left coronary artery disease [21]. It allowed to position and to work simultaneously with two 5 French-sized guide catheters at no cost of vascular-related complication (**Table 4**).

	Case 1	Case II	Case III	Case IV	Case V
Age	81	70	86	87	89
M/F	M	F	M	F	F
BMI/height (cm)/ weight (kg)	25/174/75	33/159/85	30/160/78	22/160/56	22/160/56
Frailty (0–3+)	2+	1+	3+	3+	3+
Symptoms at presentation	New chest pain and SOB CCVS Class 3	Progression of chest pain, SOB CCVS Class 3	Chest pain and SOB CCVS Class 4	Acute pulmonary edema NSTEMI VT, persistent HF	Acute pulmonary edema NSTEMI VT, persistent HF
Associated medical conditions	Severe COPD Gold IV, permanent O2 therapy	Severe COPD Gold III Past CVA and CAD	Valvular aortic stenosis, severe (< 1 cm2), COPD, transient AV block	HBP, paroxysmal atrial fibrillation Low Ef (recent)	HBP, diabetes, low Ef (recent)
CAD, syntax score (SS)	Distal LMCA Medina 1,1,1 Left dominance Syntax score 30	Distal LMCA Medina 1,1,1 Syntax score 23	distal LMCA, medina 1,1,1 occluded RCA (3VD), Syntax score 48	LMCA equivalent, 100% RCA Syntax score 28	Prox. and mid-LAD a. 75% CX a., 95% RCa. lesion 70%, syntax score 35
Addressed vessel(s)	LMCA	LMCA	LMCA	Ostial-LAD/ostial CX arteries	Prox. to distal LAD-Diag a.
Arterial access	R TUlnA/L TRA, 5F Glidesheath	R+ L TRA, 5F Glidesheath	R+ L TRA, 5F Glidesheath	R+ L TRA, 5F Glidesheath	R+ L TRA, 5F Glidesheath
Fluoroscopy time/ volume of contrast/ DAP/CPK 24 h	44′/290 ml/228 Gy/cm^2 CPK (−)	17′/212 ml/143 Gy/cm^2 CPK (−)	20′/148 ml/114 Gy/cm^2 CPK (−)	15′/140 ml/73 Gy/cm^2 CPK (−)	20′/128 ml/173 Gy/cm^2 CPK (−)
Follow-up	Alive > 1 year, acute pneumonia at 1 month	Alive > 1 year, no angina	Alive > 1 year, aortic valve stenosis said moderate	Alive > 1 year, class 1, normalized LV function	Alive > 1 year, class 1, normalized LV function (had 2 weeks re-hosp for HF)

SOB, shortness of breath; **CCVS**, Canadian Cardiovascular Society classification;

VT, ventricular tachycardia; **HF**, heart failure; **NSTEMI**, non-ST elevation myocardial infarction; **COPD**, chronic obstructive pulmonary disease (severity as assessed by the GOLD classification); **CVA**, cerebrovascular accident; **CAD**, coronary artery disease;

Ef, left ventricular ejection fraction; **LMCA**, left main coronary artery; **RCA**, right coronary artery; **3VD**, triple vessel disease; **LAD**, left anterior descending (artery); **CX**, circumflex (artery); **R TUlnA**, right transulnar artery; **L TRA**, left transradial access;

R TRA, right transradial access; **DAP**, dose area product (Gy/cm^2); **CPK**, creatine phosphokinase.

Table 4. TRA PCI and frailties, adapted from ACC, 18;3, 45-52.

6. How to avoid the radial artery occlusion problem

Coronary artery disease (CAD) is a progressive disease, and many patients "enjoying" a first successful TRA PCI will require in the future one or more interventions, evenly in emergency (subacute stent thrombosis, new STEMI or new acute coronary syndrome, etc.). So, preserving a well-patent radial artery may be lifesaving later.

In 2016, 1 year before the CRASOC studies were accepted for publication in the American Journal of Cardiology [3] as the largest randomized and prospective study analyzing the hemostasis role in radial artery occlusion (RAO). Rashid et al. published a well-documented systematic review and meta-analysis [22] about the TRA-related radial artery occlusion. It is easy to summarize the problem and to understand the different ways we must follow to reduce the RAO rate. RAO is the direct consequence of the vessel injury associated with any TRA. Injury happens at three levels, and we have to minimize the trauma at each of these levels: first, the puncture; second, the sheath insertion and catheter manipulations (within the sheath); and finally, the compression/hemostasis following the catheterization. Mention for selecting the best technique and material for artery puncture and cannulation was already made. The author makes the hope that, someday, TRA operators will get the chance to handle the specifically designed and actually patented radial artery needle: it should be the best way to reduce as far as possible the puncture-related aggression. In the same way, it is obvious that reducing the size of the sheath is another excellent way to reduce the related harm against the artery wall. Not only should the size be reduced as far as possible, but also the material must be hydrophilic: non-hydrophilic sheath should be banished from a good TRA practice. The "slippery" problem of the hydrophilic sheath is the best proof of the appropriately reduced parietal stress. This problem may be easily "fixed" at the skin level: a simple "opsite" film placed over the sheath does the job. The introduction of the Terumo® "Glidesheath" family of radial introducers represents a welcomed improvement: The company cleverly worked to offer a reduced outside diameter of the sheath (what the artery" feels") together with a normal inside diameter. It allows operators working predominantly in 5 French (including for PCI), to offer a "virtual 4F" TRA procedure for the majority of their patients.

The post-catheterization hemostasis step contributes to the global artery's damage: as proven effective thanks to the 3616 analyzed patients in the CRASOC studies, a gentle and short hemostasis with pneumatic compression (TR Band® compression device, 10 cc of air/90 minutes) represents today the best and most elegant way to minimize the RAO rate. A TRA operator has to be reminded that the hemostasis step is his last chance to save the radial artery patency.

7. Conclusion

"TRA for everybody" is highly desirable for patient safety and comfort. This strategy is achievable, and solutions for more complex populations are provided. Ways to maintain the artery patency are described. Better-suited materials for easier TRA are already offered, and innovations will continue [23, 24]. The author still believes that in year 2018 the radial way requires a gentleman attitude (at least for the radial artery), demands a rebel inclination—to discard all the negative thinking about the TRA feasibility—and is best served by a "believer" behavior: a believer always will try to find indication rather than contraindication for TRA.

Author details

Vincent Dangoisse[1,2]*

*Address all correspondence to: vdangoisse@me.com

1 CSPQ, Université de Montréal, Canada

2 Catheterization Laboratory, CIUSSS-MCQ, Hôpital Ste-Marie, Trois-Rivières, Québec, Canada

References

[1] Dangoisse V. Gentleman, rebel and believer: The radial way. Indian Heart Journal. 2010;**62**(3):202e205

[2] Saito S, Ikei H, Hosokawa G, Tanaka S. Influence of the ratio between radial artery inner diameter and sheath outer diameter on radial artery flow after transradial coronary intervention. Catheterization and Cardiovascular Interventions. 1999;**46**:173-178

[3] Dangoisse V, Guédès A, Chenu P, Hanet C, Albert C, Robin V, et al. Usefulness of a gentle and short hemostasis using the transradial band device after transradial access for percutaneous coronary angiography and interventions to reduce the radial artery occlusion rate (from the prospective and randomized CRASOC I, II, and III studies). The American Journal of Cardiology. 2017;**120**:374e379

[4] Guédès A, Dangoisse V, Gabriel L, et al. Low rate of conversion to transfemoral approach when attempting both radial arteries for coronary angiography and percutaneous coronary intervention: A study of 1,826 consecutive procedures. Journal of Invasive Cardiology. 2010;**22**(9):391-397

[5] Dangoisse V, Guédès A. Radial artery cannulation and transradial access for percutaneous coronary angiography and interventions: From experience to expertise of a single cardiac centre. J Anesthe Clinic Res. 2012;**4**:322. DOI: 10.4172/2155-6148.1000322

[6] Dangoisse V. Vascular Needle System 2016; United States Patent, No.: US 9,408,999 B2, Date of Patent: Aug 9

[7] Dangoisse V. Vascular Needle System, JPN, Patent, No.: 6043301, Date of Patent: Nov 18, 2016

[8] Fernandez et al. Safety and efficacy of ulnar artery approach for percutaneous cardiac catheterization: Systematic review and meta-analysis. Catheterization and Cardiovascular Interventions. 2018;**91**:1273-1280

[9] Nilsson T, Lagerqvist B, Tornvall P. Coronary angiography of patients with a previous coronary by-pass operation is associated with a three times increased risk for neurological complications. A report from the Swedish Coronary Angiography and Angioplasty Registry (SCAAR). Scandinavian Cardiovascular Journal. 2009;**43**(6):374-379

[10] Louvard Y. Graft angiography via the right transradial approach. In: Marco J, Fajadet J, editors. Endovascular Therapy Course Coronary and Peripheral: Ninth Complex Coronary Angioplasty Course Book. Paris: Europa Edition; 1998. pp. 325-327

[11] Yabe J, Hirose Y, Kouchi N, Ohmura M, Lijima S, Tanaka K, et al. Is LIMA angiography possible with right radial approach? The use of left Judkins 1.0 (BABY Judkins). Japanese Journal of Interventional Cardiology. 1998;**13**(Suppl I):169

[12] Kim MH, Cha KS, Kim HJ, Kim JS. Bilateral selective internal mammary artery angiography via right radial approach: Clinical experience with newly designed Yumiko catheter. Catheterization and Cardiovascular Interventions. 2001;**54**:19-24

[13] Cha KS, Kim MH. Feasibility and safety of concomitant left internal mammary arteriography at the setting of the right transradial coronary angiography. Catheterization and Cardiovascular Interventions. 2002;**56**:188-195

[14] Sanmartin M, Cuevas D, Moxica J, Valdes M, Esparza J, Baz JA, et al. Transradial cardiac catheterization in patients with coronary bypass grafts: Feasibility analysis and comparison with transfemoral approach. Catheterization and Cardiovascular Interventions. 2006;**67**:580-584

[15] Burzotta F, Trani C, Hamon M, Amoroso G, Kiemeneij F. Transradial approach for coronary angiography and interventions in patients with coronary bypass grafts: Tips and tricks. Catheterization and Cardiovascular Interventions. 2008;**72**:263-272

[16] Rathore S, Roberts E, Hakeem AR, Pauriah M, Beaumont A, Morris JL. The feasibility of percutaneous transradial coronary intervention for saphenous vein graft lesions and comparison with transfemoral route. Journal of Interventional Cardiology. 2009;**22**:336-340

[17] Caputo RP, Tremmel JA, Rao S, Gilchrist IC, Pyne C, Pancholy S, et al. Transradial arterial access for coronary and peripheral procedures: Executive summary by the transradial committee of the SCAI. Catheterization and Cardiovascular Interventions. 2011;**78**(6):823-839

[18] Dangoisse V, Guédès A, Gabriel L, Jamart J, Marchandise B, Chenu P, et al. Transradial approach for evaluation of post Coronary Artery Bypass Graft surgery patients: Left or Right radial artery when both mammary arteries are grafted? Journal of the American College of Cardiology. 2012;**59**(13s1):E187-E187. DOI: 10.13140/2.1.3654.1440

[19] Dangoisse V, Guédès A, Gabriel L, Jamart J, Chenu P, Marchandise B, et al. Full conversion from transfemoral to transradial approach for percutaneous coronary interventions results in a similar success rate and a rapid reduction of in-hospital cardiac and vascular major events. EuroIntervention. 2013;**9**:345e352

[20] Mehran R, Pocock SJ, Nikolsky E, Clayton T, Dangoas GD, Kirtane AJ, et al. A risk score to predict bleeding in patients with acute coronary syndromes. Journal of the American College of Cardiology. 2010;**55**:2556-2566. DOI: 10.1016/j.jacc.2009.09.076

[21] Dangoisse V, Schroeder E, Hanet C, Guédès A, Pancholy S. Double guide double wrist 5F left coronary artery transradial percutaneous coronary intervention and the X-Kiss technique. Acute Cardiac Care. 2017;**18**(3):45-52. DOI: 10.1080/17482941.2017.1369126 (http://www.tandfonline.com/doi/full/10.1080/17482941.2017.1369126)

[22] Rashid M, Kwok CS, Pancholy S, Chugh S, Kedev SA, Bernat I, et al. Radial artery occlusion after transradial interventions: A systematic review and meta-analysis. Journal of the American Heart Association. 2016;**5**:e002686

[23] Dangoisse V. New 6F guiding catheter for right transradial RCA-percutaneous coronary interventions: First report of performance. JACC: Cardiovascular Interventions. 2013;**6**(2_S):S27. DOI: 10.1016/j.jcin.2012.12.098

[24] Dangoisse V. A new 5F guiding catheter for right transradial LCA-percutaneous coronary interventions: First report of performance. Catheterization and Cardiovascular Interventions. 2013;**81**(S1):S93-94-D024. DOI: 10.1002/ ccd.24919

Chapter 3

The Role of Catheter Reshaping at the Angiographic Success

Yakup Balaban

Additional information is available at the end of the chapter

http://dx.doi.org/10.5772/intechopen.79210

Abstract

In coronary angiography, inability to selectively visualize anomalous coronary arteries is one of the major problems, which a cardiologist encounters during angiography. The process we expect to finish in 15 min can take hours. The angiography times exceeding 1 h are not uncommon. On 2.6% of coronary angiograms, anomalous origin of coronary arteries is encountered. In 0.58% of the cases, the left anterior descending artery (LAD) arises from a separate ostium. The absence of the left main coronary artery (LMCA) can be discerned directly on coronary angiograms obtained using selective visualization of the left circumflex (Cx) or LAD because in most of the cases, the LAD and circumflex artery (Cx) arise from separate ostia. In such situations and where it seems impossible to achieve imaging of anomalous coronary artery, catheter reshaping can be accepted as a solution. This method can be used looking for the carotid and vertebral arteries at the angiography performed via the radial or femoral route also the right and left coronary ostia with anomalous origin, that easily and safely.

Keywords: catheter reshaping, angiographic success, anomalous coronary origins

1. Coronary anomalies and frequency

For arteries that cannot be selectively visualized frequently, the presence of anomalous origins is looked for, and if they cannot be displayed for the second time, diagnosis of single or atresic coronary arteries is made [1–5]. The most common coronary artery abnormalities are follows; the right coronary artery (RCA) arising from a superoanterior position or left coronary sinus (0.65%), the LAD and Cx arising from separate ostia (0.48%), the Cx arising from the right coronary ostium (0.20%), the LAD arising from the right coronary sinus (0.20%), the single coronary artery is the LMCA (0.02%), the single coronary artery is the RCA (0.11%), and the

LAD arising from the pulmonary artery (0.02%, ALPACA syndrome). The LAD originated from the LIMA can also be present rarely in cases (Balaban Syndrome) (**Figures 1** and **2** and **Table 1**). In most of these cases during angiography, standard catheters fail to selectively visualize the anomalous coronary arteries [1–4] (**Figures 1** and **2** and **Table 1**).

In publications on anomalous origins and their incidence rates, detection of anomaly has been made in autopsy or using computed tomography. Currently, there are no encountered

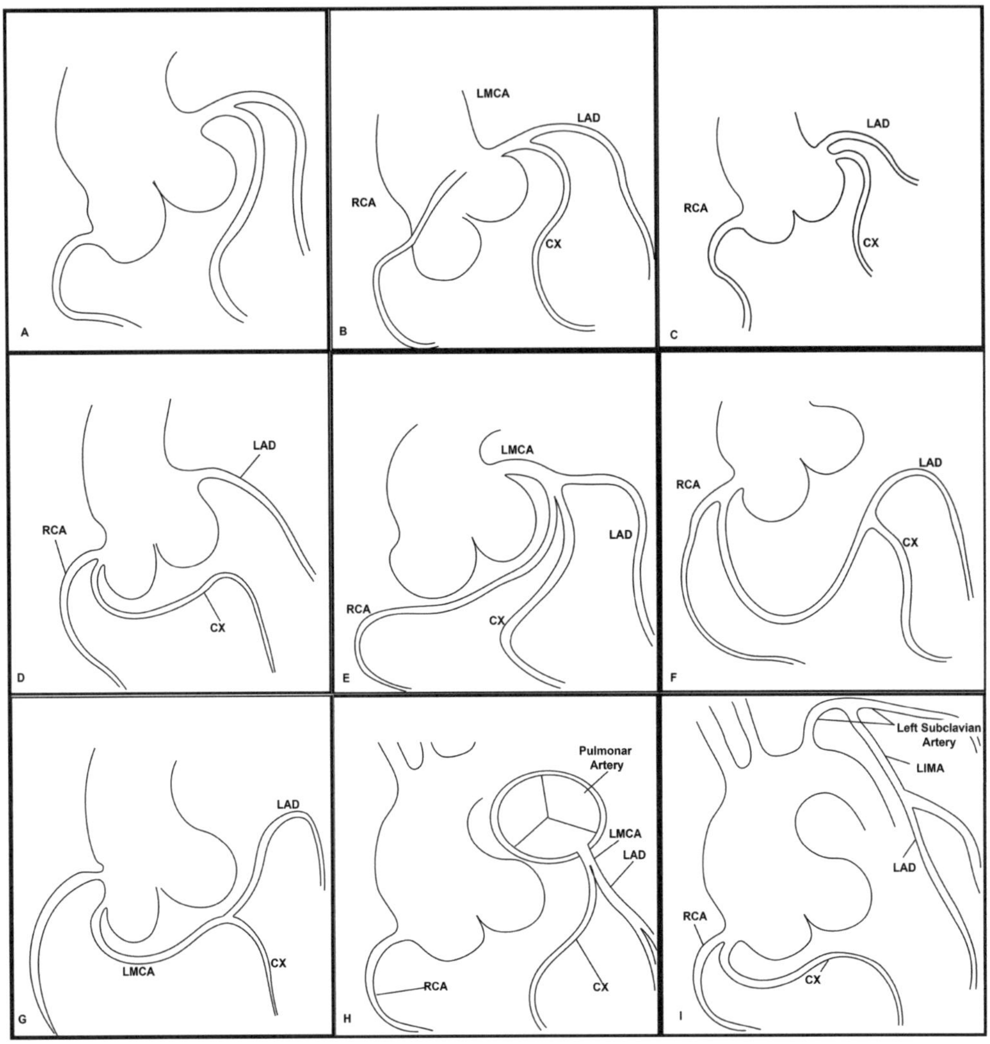

Figure 1. (A) Normal variation is 97.4% of the population. (B) The RCA arising from a superoanterior position or left coronary sinus (0.65%). (C) The LAD and Cx arising from separate ostia (0.48%). (D) The Cx arising from the right coronary ostium (0.20%). (E) The single coronary artery is the LMCA (0.02%). (F) The single coronary artery is the right coronary artery (0.11%). (G) The LAD arising from the right coronary sinus (0.20%). (H) The LAD arising from the pulmonary artery is a very rarely encountered anomaly (0.02% ALPACA syndrome). (I) The LAD is originated from LIMA in the very rarely encountered cases.

http://dx.doi.org/10.5772/intechopen.79210

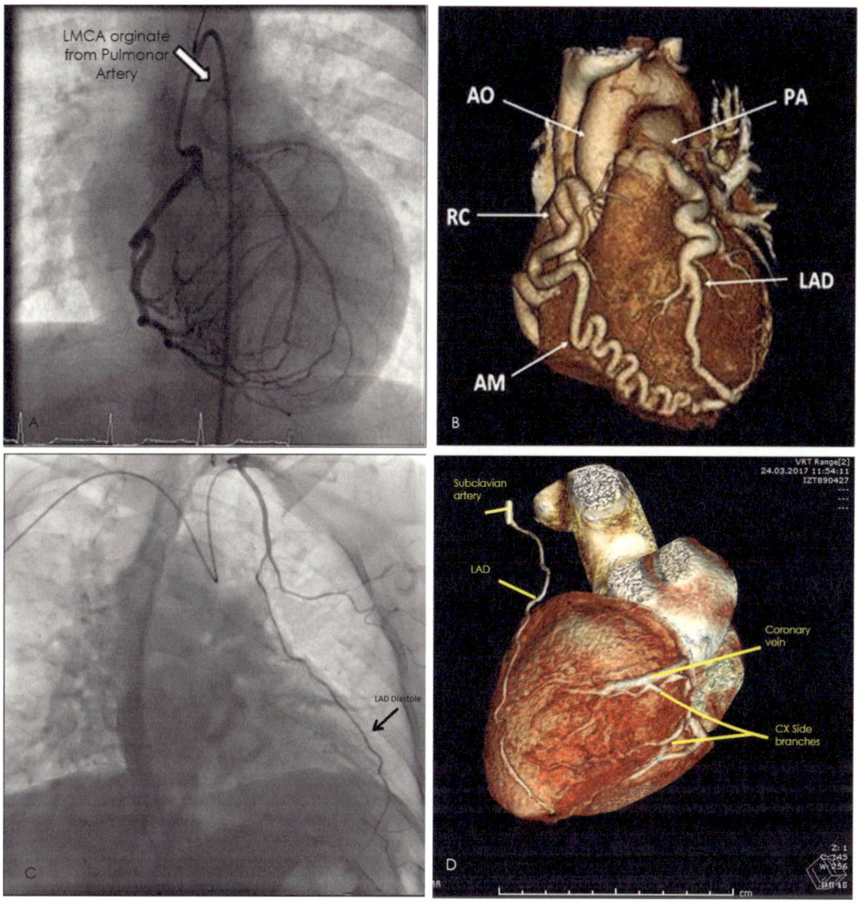

Figure 2. (A, B) The LAD arising from the pulmonary artery is a very rarely encountered anomaly (0.02% ALPACA syndrome). (C, D) The LAD is originated from the LIMA in the very rarely encountered cases (Balaban Syndrome).

comprehensive and detailed publications related to angiographically defined coronary arteries of anomalous origin or their incidence. In patients with anomalous coronary arteries, by shaping catheter, angiographic visualization of anomalous coronary arteries may be enabled within a short time and using lesser amount of opaque material [6–8].

If the physician does not suspect the presence of another coronary artery, this negligence may lead to catastrophic consequences during a potential attack of myocardial infarction in cases with anomalous origin of coronary arteries, inability to visualize the coronary artery [6].

In nearly 97.4% of the patient population, selective visualization of coronary arteries can be achieved with the aid of catheters available in most of the catheterization laboratories. However, in the remaining 2.6% of the cases, these catheters cannot aid in visualization. Otherwise, if an infarction-related coronary artery could not be selectively detected, this condition may lead to fatal consequences for the patient [1–8].

Anomalous origin	Incidence (%)
High take off RCA or from left CS (**Figure 1B**)	0.65
LAD and CX arising from separate ostia (**Figure 1C**)	0.48
CX arising from right CS (**Figure 1D**)	0.20
Single coronary artery RCA (**Figure 1E**)	0.11
Single coronary artery LMCA(**Figure 1F**)	0.02
LAD arising from the right coronary sinus (**Figure 1G**)	0.20
LAD arising from pulmonary artery(**Figure 1H**)	0.02
LAD arising from LIMA(**Figure 1I**)	0.001

Coronary arteries of anomalous origin, and their incidence rates. LAD: left anterior descending artery; CX: circumflex artery; RCA: right coronary artery; LMCA: left main coronary artery; CS: coronary sinus.

Table 1. Incidence rates of coronary arteries of anomalous origin.

In these circumstances a physician who is both an explorer and an inventor in cases of MI may save the life of his/her patient.

In cases with coronary arteries with anomalous origin, which are difficult or even impossible to visualize in catheterization laboratory, after determination of approximate origin and angle of exit of the coronary artery, it is possible to design a catheter that can negotiate anomalous origin and angle of exit. Shaping catheter may be an effective, reliable, and in cases with acute MI, life-saving procedure in the achievement of visualization and decreasing the duration of the procedure, radiation dose, and opaque material used [4, 8].

2. The catheter reshaping method

The standard diagnostic catheters that we use in angiography can be reshaped with the standardized methods that we explain as below:

The distal tip of the 0.035 inch guidewire that we use during angiography is inserted through the distal tip of the catheter and advanced for 10 cm. Then, with the aid of the guidewire, the required shaping can be performed. Afterwards, the end of the catheter is held 10 cm away from a heat gun and exposed to hot air (450°C) for 4–6 s. Soon after the tip of the heated and reshaped catheter is immersed in water. Using a plastic injector, the catheter with the guidewire inside is irrigated from the opposite end using a sterile isotonic saline solution. Before completion of the cooling process, the guidewire is removed, and water cooling is continued. When the catheter is completely cooled, the catheter is cannulated with the aid of a 0.38-inch guidewire using rotational movements through the carotid ostium or anomalous coronary ostium to visualize the carotid or coronary arteries (**Figures 3** and **4**) [4, 8–12].

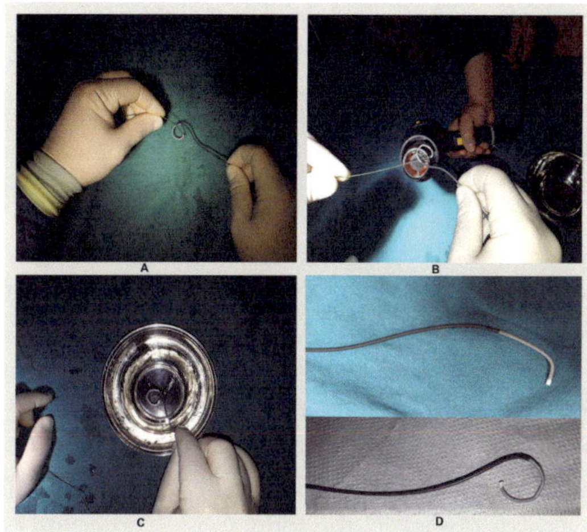

Figure 3. The catheter reshaping method for carotid angiography via transradial approach: (A) the distal tip of the 0.035 inch guidewire we used during angiography was inserted through the distal tip of the catheter and advanced for 10 cm. With the aid of the guidewire, the required shaping was then performed. (B) Afterwards, the end of the catheter was held 10 cm away from a heat gun and exposed to hot air (450°C) for 4–6 s. Soon after the tip of the heated and reshaped catheter was immersed in water. (C) Using a plastic injector, the catheter with the guidewire inside was irrigated from the opposite end using a sterile isotonic saline solution. Before completion of the cooling process, the guidewire was removed, and water cooling was continued. (D) Final viewing of the reshaped catheter.

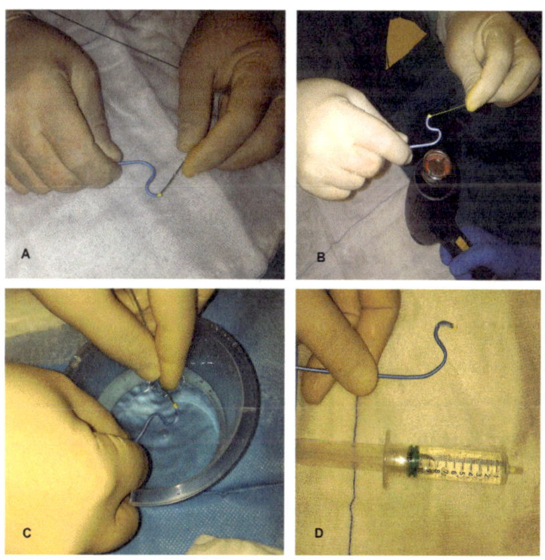

Figure 4. The catheter reshaping for carotid angiography via femoral way: (A) the distal tip of the 0.035 inch guidewire we used during angiography was inserted through the distal tip of the catheter and advanced for 10 cm. With the aid of the guidewire, the required shaping was then performed. (B) Afterwards, the end of the catheter was held 10 cm away from a heat gun and exposed to hot air (450°C) for 4–6 s. Soon after the tip of the heated and reshaped catheter was immersed in water. (C) Using a plastic injector, the catheter with the guidewire inside was irrigated from the opposite end using a sterile isotonic saline solution. Before completion of the cooling process, the guidewire was removed, and water cooling was continued. (D) Final viewing of the reshaped catheter.

3. Types of aortic arches and their incidence rates

In cases where selective angiography is not successful, it is necessary to know the anomaly in order to solve the problem. The identification of aortic type may be helpful to determine the most appropriate shape of catheter. At first, the physician should know and form an estimate aortic arch and coronary origin anatomy.

In some publications, various classifications for various types of aortic arches have been proposed. Most of such classification schemes fail to improve the transradial angiography procedure. We have recently proposed a classification system. Type I aortic arches, also known as normal aortic arches, are the most frequently encountered (86%). In this arch type, the right carotid artery arises from the right brachial trunk, and the left common carotid artery originates from the aortic arch 1–2 cm to the left of the brachiocephalic trunk. In 9% of cases in which a Type II aortic arch is observed, the right and left common carotid arteries originate from the brachial trunk. In Type III aortic arches (2%), the right and left common carotid arteries directly originate from the aortic arch as a one unit or separately. In Type IV aortic arches (3%), which also include arteria lusoria, the right subclavian artery stems from the aorta near the descending aorta after the carotid arteries [9, 10, 13–15] (**Figure 5**).

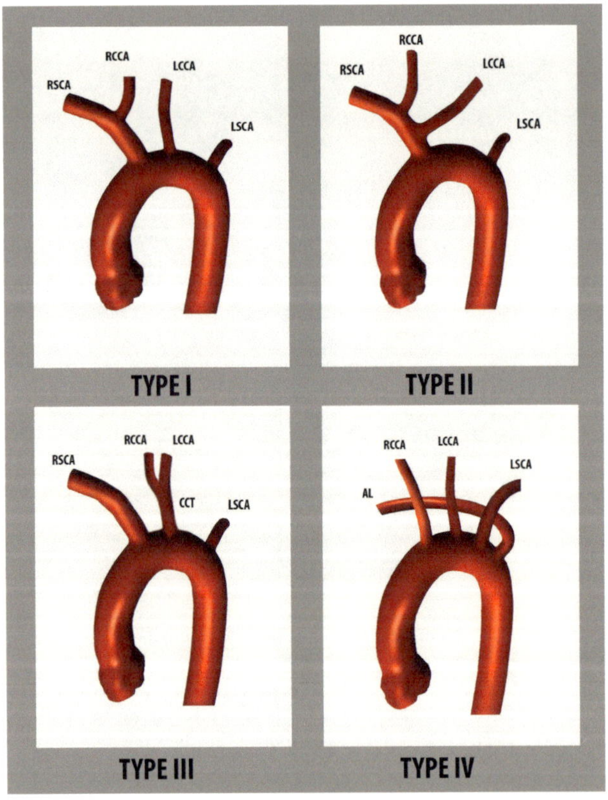

Figure 5. RSCA, right subclavian artery; LCCA, left common carotid artery; RCCA, left common carotid artery; LSCA, left subclavian artery. Types I, II, III, and IV are encountered in 86, 9, 2, and 3% of cases, respectively.

4. The role of catheter reshaping in the success of carotid angiography by radial pathway

It is difficult to perform transradial carotid angiography using conventional multipurpose catheters, which suffer from lower success rates and longer procedural times. Therefore, physicians do not prefer to perform transradial carotid angiography. We thought that among conventional catheters, the Simpson catheter and the 3.5 JL catheter were the most suitable for transradial visualization. To this end, the reshaped catheters can be more effective than available conventional catheters in carotid angiography. There are a few new publications in this regard, reaching 1500 participants. However, one study has examined the use of the modified Simmons catheter in the right transradial route carotid angiography. The Simpson catheter has an angled distal tip, which opens far from the long axis of the catheter. This configuration decreases the right transradial procedural success rate of selective visualization of the left carotid artery in cases where the left carotid artery stems from a point near the brachiocephalic trunk. Therefore, performing selective angiography with a Simpson catheter requires special experience and manual dexterity. The retroflexed tip of the 3.5 JL catheter provides improved cannulation of the left common carotid artery and is one of the most frequently available catheters in every laboratory [9–11, 16].

Even though transradial carotid visualization can be achieved using standard catheters, carotid arteries cannot be selectively cannulated, and the images obtained are far from satisfactory

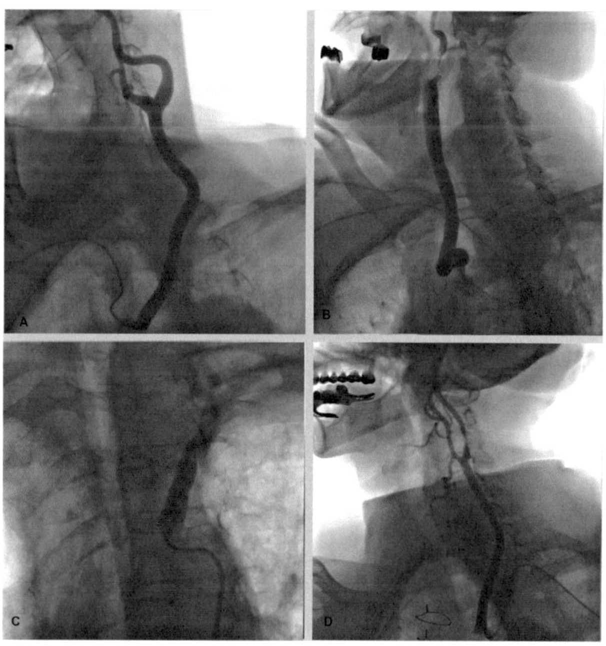

Figure 6. The reshaped catheter types using at the different angiographies: (A) right transradial carotid angiography with hooklike reshaped catheter; (B) the right transradial carotid angiography in the arteria lusoria case (type IV aorta); (C) the "S"-shaped catheter using with femoral access; and (D) the left transradial carotid angiography with the "hooklike" reshaped catheter.

compared with the selective images. The size and track of the plaque, in particular, cannot be clearly evaluated. Only the degree of stenosis may be estimated. However, determining the morphology and fragility of the plaque, and the presence of vascularity or plaque dissection and erosion, is required to predict the probability of experiencing a cerebrovascular event in the future and for planning the appropriate treatment modality and decreasing procedural complications. The new visualization method that is catheter reshaping is more useful to detect the presence of plaque fractures, erosion, and dissection due to good quality images. These satisfactory images aid us in selection of appropriate treatment methods and prediction of complications [10] (**Figure 6**).

The visualization with new reshaped catheter requires a shorter procedural time and less opaque material usage. Since selective engagement of catheters in carotid arteries is achieved with this method, higher-quality images can be obtained. The new catheter greatly contributes to the determination of appropriate treatment [10, 17].

5. Following coronary angiography performed by femoral approach, the carotid angiography, and the contribution of the catheter reshape to success

The relationship between peripheral artery disease and coronary artery disease is a known fact. This relationship is often predictive of stroke, renal insufficiency, and extremity artery disease in patients with coronary artery disease. At the moment of coronary angiography procedure, the visualisable of carotids seems to be advantageous for the patient. The carotids can be displayed noninvasively by MR angiography and CT angiography. But it can only be displayed at low resolution according to invasive angiography. This noninvasive imaging may be the first choice, for isolated cases. However, in patients already undergoing coronary angiography, carotid imaging application following this procedure is a more appropriate choice. The quality of the invasive carotid image is still better than the MR and CT angiography. Invasive imaging is still the gold standard in neck malformations, carotid tumors, neck injuries, and carotid artery stenosis. In still today, cardiovascular surgeons, neurologists, and neurosurgeons, if they see lesions in the carotid artery at the MR and CT angiography, require invasive carotid angiography when they propose an additional intervention for these lesions [9, 10, 12–18].

It is known that physicians who perform coronary angiography use "the right diagnostic catheter" for their desired carotid imaging. Simon catheters and HN4–5, CK1, and MAN catheters can be used, especially if carotid interventional procedures are going to be performed. However, these catheters are not commonly used by cardiologists. They can often be supplied by special order, and they are not available in most coronary angiography laboratories. For these reasons, the reshaping of catheter in the coronary angiography laboratory can be a snapshot solution to the problem of imaging anomalous vascular origins and for carotid and other peripheral arterial imaging [4, 9, 10, 12, 19–21]. There is a strong relationship between carotid artery disease and coronary artery disease. According to recent studies, in patients with coronary artery stenosis of 50% or more, the likelihood of a significant carotid artery stenosis exceeds 60%. This ratio can be interpreted; if carotid angiography is performed in the patients with a significant coronary stenosis, carotid artery disease can be shown at least among 60% of the patients. Therefore, in patients with planned coronary angiography, it would be useful to look at carotids in in the presence of severe coronary atherosclerosis at the same session without preliminary investigation of carotid stenosis. Also the opposite can also be considered. In other words, that is very useful to perform coronary angiography at the same procedure in the patient with carotid stenosis. At least 60% of these patients with carotid artery disease have also significant coronary artery disease [9, 10, 20–22].

In the patients with carotid stenosis by Doppler ultrasonography, invasive angiography may be more advantageous than MR and CT angiography, because if a person has carotid stenosis, there is a high probability of coronary artery disease. If we focus on carotid stenosis and ignore potential coronary artery disease, the patient may become vulnerable to myocardial infarction. Furthermore, the image quality of noninvasive techniques is not as detailed as in the invasive angiography. The conventional angiography can show the character of carotid plaque, the cracks in the plaque, whether the plaque is vulnerable or not. Knowing plaque features give valuable information to physicians for treatment approach [9, 10, 18–27].

Cardiologists who perform carotid angiography followed by coronary angiography perform carotid angiography often with the right Judkins diagnostic catheter. There are no clinical studies conducted to determine which of the HN4-5, CK1, and MAN catheters are more effective and reliable in carotid angiography [21, 22]. The cardiologists performing coronary angiography can make a very successful and reliable carotid angiography by giving the "S" shape to "right diagnostic catheter" at the transfemoral way or by giving "hooklike" shape to right diagnostic catheter at the transradial way, without having an additional catheter in the catheterization laboratory (**Figures 3, 4,** and **6**) [9, 10].

Catheter shaping is done as an amateur in many coronary angiography laboratories. There are clinical trials that standardize catheter reshaping. The reliability and success of catheter shaping by hand have been proven with these clinical studies reaching over 1500 participants. Teaching and implementing this method in daily practice may be useful [9, 10, 12, 17].

All experiences and discoveries are creating new percutaneous intervention areas. Twenty years ago, transcatheter aortic valve replacement was a dream. The retrograde chronic total occlusion intervention was almost impossible with techniques and instruments of 15 years ago. All these developments have been made possible by the transformation of new methods into scientific publications [28, 29].

The initial experience of angiography was performed with brachial pathway, but the femoral route was considered safer and simpler at the beginning. Therefore, the development of angiography has been initiated using the femoral route. However, in the last 15 years, radial route has been used again and even has been shown to have advantages, so it is used now all over the world. Today, coronary and peripheral invasive angiography can be performed as fast and reliable as MR and CT angiography. Invasive angiography allows for real-time imaging and immediate intervention allowing physicians to better identify condition of patient and treatment of the disease. All interventional physicians should strive to publish the useful and practical methods that they have recently discovered. These publications are very important because they can shed light on the development of new techniques and devices [30–32] (**Figures 3, 4,** and **6**).

6. Conclusion

The newly obtained catheter by reshaping of the plastic catheters used in angiography by cooling after reshaping with heat can be more effective at the displaying vessels with anomalous origin than existing catheters. First, the aortography must be performed to determine the location of the coronary artery ostium in the aorta at the anomalous coronary events. Thus, the appropriate catheter shape can be estimated. The selective angiography can be quite easy if the current catheter can be successfully shaped. This method can also be used to image the carotid and vertebral arteries by radial and femoral routes. The carotid and vertebral artery angiography can be performed more easily with the use of reshaped catheters in some cases including anomalous coronary cases.

Author details

Yakup Balaban

Address all correspondence to: yakupbalaban@gmail.com

Department of Cardiology, VM Medical Park Kocaeli Hospital, Turkey

References

[1] Graidis C, Dimitriadis D, Karasavvidis V, Dimitriadis G, Argyropoulou E, et al. Prevalence and characteristics of coronary artery anomalies in an adult population undergoing multidetector-row computed tomography for the evaluation of coronary artery disease. BMC Cardiovascular Disorders. 2015;**15**:112

[2] Mavi A, Ayalp R, Serçelik A, Pesţemalci T, Batyraliev T, Gümüşburun E. Frequency of the anomalous origin of the left main coronary artery with angiography in a Turkish population. Acta Medica Okayama. 2004;**58**(1):17-22

[3] Ayalp R, Mavi A, Serçelik A, Batyraliev T, Gümüsburun E. Frequency of the anomalous origin of the right coronary artery with angiography in a Turkish population. International Journal of Cardiology. 2002;**82**(3):253-257

[4] Balaban YHA, Gümrükçüoğlu D, Güngör SC. Left anterior descending artery of anomalous origin; native LAD arises from left internal mammarian artery. A case report and article review. Cardiovascular Revascularization Medicine. 2018;**19**(2):209-214

[5] Villa AD, Sammut E, Nair A, Rajani R, Bonamini R, Chiribiri A. Coronary artery anomalies overview: The normal and the abnormal. World Journal of Radiology. 2016;**8**(6):537-555

[6] Frescura C, Basso C, Thiene G, Corrado D, Pennelli T, et al. Anomalous origin of coronary arteries and risk of sudden death: A study based on an autopsy population of congenital heart disease. Human Pathology. 1998;**29**(7):689-695

[7] Gräni C, Benz DC, Schmied C, Vontobel J, Possner M, et al. Prevalence and characteristics of coronary artery anomalies detected by coronary computed tomography angiography in 5634 consecutive patients in a single Centre in Switzerland. Swiss Medical Weekly. 2016;**146**:w14294

[8] Kim JY, Yoon GS, Doh HJ, Choe HM, Kwon SU, Namgung J. Two cases of successful primary percutaneous coronary intervention in patients with an anomalous right coronary artery arising from the left coronary cusp. Korean Circulation Journal. 2008;**38**(3):179-183

[9] Balaban Y. New developed femoral-S carotid catheter' is very effective and safe in carotid angiography: A retrospective study OMICS. Journal of Radiology. 2017;**6**:6

[10] Balaban Y. Effectiveness of a handmade "new carotid catheter" in transradial carotid angiography: A comparison with conventional multipurpose catheters. Journal of Interventional Cardiology. 2018;**31**(1):94-105. DOI: 10.1111/joic.12454. Epub: October 11, 2017

[11] Cha KS, Kim MH, Kim YD, Kim JS. Combined right transradial coronary angiography and selective carotid angiography: Safety and feasibility in unselected patients. Catheterization and Cardiovascular Interventions. 2001;**53**(3):380-385

[12] Erden I, Golcuk E, Bozyel S, Erden EC, Balaban Y, Yalın K, et al. Effectiveness of handmade "Jacky-like catheter" As a single multipurpose catheter in transradial coronary angiography: A randomized comparison with conventional two-catheter strategy. Journal of Interventional Cardiology. 2017;**30**(1):24-32

[13] Huapaya JA, Trujillo KC, Trelles M, Carbaja RD, Espadin RF. Anatomic variations of the branches of the aortic arch in a Peruvian population. Medwave. 2015;**15**(6):e6194. DOI: 10.5867/medwave.2015.06.6194

[14] Ergun E, Simsek B, Kosar P, Yilmaz BK, Turgut AT. Anatomical variations in branching patterns of arcus aorta: 64-slice CTA appearance. Surgical and Radiologic Anatomy. 2014;**36**(10):1105-1106. DOI: 10.1007/s00276-014-1288-4. Epub: March 27, 2014

[15] Cummings MS, Kuo BT, Ziada KM. A rare anomaly of the aortic arch: Aberrant right subclavian artery associated with common carotid trunk. The Journal of Invasive Cardiology. 2011;**23**(10):E241-E243

[16] Park JH, Kim DY, Kim JW, Park YS, Seung WB. Efficacy of transradial cerebral angiography in the elderly. Journal of Korean Neurosurgical Association. 2013;**53**(4):213-217. DOI: 10.3340/jkns.2013.53.4.213. Epub: April 30, 2013

[17] Fang Y, Yang C, Wang X, Zhou L, Wang H, Zeng C. Feasibility and application of single 5F multipurpose catheter in coronary and peripheral angiography via a transradial approach. International Journal of Cardiology. 2011;**151**:182-118

[18] Ledwoch J, Staubach S, Segerer M, Strohm H, Mudra H. Incidence and risk factors of embolized particles in carotid artery stenting and association with clinical outcome. International Journal of Cardiology. 2017;**227**:550-555. DOI: 10.1016/j.ijcard.2016.10.103. Epub: November 2, 2016

[19] Rafailidis V, Chryssogonidis I, Tegos T, Kouskouras K, Charitanti-Kouridou A. Imaging of the ulcerated carotid atherosclerotic plaque: A review of the literature. Insights into Imaging. 2017;**8**(2):213-225. DOI: 10.1007/s13244-017-0543-8

[20] Rigatelli G. Screening angiography of supraaortic vessels performed by invasive cardiologists at the time of cardiac catheterization: Indications and results. The International Journal of Cardiovascular Imaging. 2005;**21**(2-3):179-183

[21] Seo WK, Yong HS, Koh SB, Suh SI, Kim JH, Yu SW, et al. Correlation of coronary artery atherosclerosis with atherosclerosis of the intracranial cerebral artery and the extracranial carotid artery. European Neurology. 2008;**59**(6):292-298. DOI: 10.1159/000121418. Epub: April 11, 2008

[22] Bae HJ, Yoon BW, Kang DW, Koo JS, Lee SH, Kim KB, et al. Correlation of coronary and cerebral atherosclerosis: Difference between extracranial and intracranial arteries. Cerebrovascular Diseases. 2006;**21**(1-2):112-119. Epub: December 9, 2005

[23] Rigatelli G, Gemelli M, Zamboni A, Docali G, Rossi P, Grazio M. Significance of selective carotid angiography during complete cardiac catheterization in patients candidates to combined aortic valve and carotid surgery. Minerva Cardioangiologica. 2003;**51**(3):305-309

[24] Rigatelli G. Diagnosis of carotid artery occlusive disease in patients scheduled for cardiac or vascular surgery: Is this a place for invasive selective carotid angiography? Stroke. 2004;**35**(5):e89-e90; Author reply: e89-90. Epub: March 25, 2004

[25] Korotkikh NG, Ol'shanskiĭ MS, Stepanov IV. Multidisciplinary approach to diagnostics of extensive vascular head and neck malformations. Stomatologiia (Mosk). 2012;**91**(1):40-45

[26] Korotkikh NG, Ol'shanskiĭ MS, Stepanov IV, Mashkova TA, Nerovnyĭ AI, Panchenko IG. The multidisciplinary approach to diagnostics and treatment of hypervascular masses in ENTstructures. Vestnik Otorinolaringologii. 2013;**5**:44-47

[27] Arslan F1, Yılmaz S, Özer F, Andıç C, Canpolat T, Yavuz H. Surgical treatment of carotid body tumors. Kulak Burun Boğaz Ihtisas Dergisi. 2013;**23**(6):336-340. DOI: 10.5606/kbbihtisas.2013.28159

[28] Kaneda H, Takahashi S, Saito S. Successful coronary intervention for chronic total occlusion in an anomalous right coronary artery using the retrograde approach via a collateral vessel. The Journal of Invasive Cardiology. 2007;**19**(1):E1-E4

[29] Cribier A, Eltchaninoff H, Tron C, Bauer F, Agatiello C. Early experience with percutaneous transcatheter implantation of heart valve prosthesis for the treatment of end-stage inoperable patients with calcific aortic stenosis. Journal of the American College of Cardiology. 2004;**43**(4):698-703

[30] Morgan JH, Johnson JH, Brown RB, Harvey RL, Rizzoni WE, Tyson CS. Initial experience with routine selective carotid arteriography by vascular surgeons. The American Surgeon. 2006;**72**(8):684-686; Discussion 687

[31] Louvard Y, Lefèvre T, Allain A, Morice M. Coronary angiography through the radial or the femoral approach: The CARAFE study. Catheterization and Cardiovascular Interventions. 2001;**52**(2):181-187

[32] Oren O, Oren M, Turgeman Y. Transradial versus Transfemoral approach in peripheral arterial interventions. International Journal of Angiology. 2016;**25**(3):148-152. DOI: 10.1055/s-0035-1563607. Epub: September 7, 2015

Chapter 4

Stent's Manufacturing Field: Past, Present, and Future Prospects

Antonio J. Guerra and Joaquim Ciurana

Additional information is available at the end of the chapter

http://dx.doi.org/10.5772/intechopen.81668

Abstract

From the introduction of stents, nobody was able to predict the advances that will occur in stent technology over the upcoming decades. Since their appearances, it became evident that this device had significant limitations, such as vessel occlusion and/or restenosis. Despite that, this medical device is the best clinical solution for cardiovascular vessel occlusions. Stents require a deep analysis, in terms of thrombogenicity, manufacturing process, geometrical aspects, and mechanical performance, among many other characteristics. The surface quality obtained in their manufacture process is crucial to blood compatibility, prevents the activation process of thrombosis, and improves the healing efficiency. The forecast stent market makes necessary continuous studies on this field, which help to solve the medical and engineering problems of this device, which are in constant development. Stents have been the center of many research lines over the last decades. The present chapter aims to summarize the state of the art of this medical device in the last years in the fields of design, manufacturing, and materials.

Keywords: stent, BMS, DES, BRS, ETS, permanent, fully absorbable, design, FEA, manufacturing, processes, material

1. Introduction

In medicine, atherosclerotic vascular diseases are common and life-threatening diseases that narrows the vessels and reduces the blood flow in the arteries. Nowadays, angioplasty, also known as percutaneous coronary intervention (PCI), or peripheral artery balloon dilation and stenting are frequently used interventional therapeutic methods, in which a special tubing (stent) is usually placed to open the narrowed arterial vessel.

From the introduction of PCI, nobody was able to predict the advances that will occur in stent technology over the upcoming decades [1]. Since PCI appearances, it became evident that this approach has significant limitations, such as vessel occlusion and/or restenosis [2]. To overcome these problems, bare metal stents (BMS) were introduced, and despite reducing the vessel occlusion, however, high rates of restenosis constituted their major limitation [3]. To surmount this hurdle, the metallic stent coated with antiproliferative drug was conceived, the drug-eluting stents (DES). With the introduction of DES, the antiproliferative drug over the struts prolonged vessel wall healing, reduced neointima hyperplasia, and consequently decreased the target lesion revascularization (TLR). The most important limitation of the first generation of DES was related to the lack of biocompatibility of the drug-eluting polymer leading to a persistent inflammatory response after the drug-eluting period. Although permanent stents (BMS and DES) are effective, in most cases, the role of stent is temporary and is limited to the intervention, and shortly thereafter, until healing and re-endothelialization are obtained [4]. Bioresorbable stents (BRS) were introduced to overcome these limitations with important advantages: complete bioresorption, mechanical flexibility, etc. The BRS concept introduced the use of polymers in stenting procedures for the first time. With the inclusion of polymeric materials in the field of stents, a new and promising idea makes its way, electrospun tubular scaffolds (ETS) for stenting process. Unlike current stents, ETS theoretically could present some advances such as (I) better longitudinal flexibility to help the placement of the stent and (II) their surface mimics body tissue to help to obtain a best proliferation rates [5] and thus a rapid endothelialization. Nevertheless, ETS could have some disadvantages such as their radial flexibility. The radial expansion of ETS will occur by elongation of its fibers, in contrast to current stents in which it occurs by elongation of its radial cells. This fact could make correct vessel support difficult, which would restrict the use of ETS for only peripheral applications. With the author's best knowledge, this new idea has been overlooked, but it presents a promising approach to solve cardiovascular problems.

Stents can be used for a wide range of indication: de novo lesions, small vessel disease (SVD), bifurcation lesions, and tortuous and narrows lesions. Stents can improve the clinical outcomes for all of these indications as well as quality of life for patients suffering from this debilitating disease. In 2013, sales of DES and BMS in the 10 major markets were $ 4.89 billion. Global data [6] estimates that by 2020, sales of stents will grow to $ 5.65 billion.

2. Stent manufacturing process design

Regardless of the stent choice, BMS, DES, BRS, or ETS, the challenges associated to this medical device remain similar. **Figure 1** shows the *pyramid of stent manufacturing process design*. It represents the main issues to consider at the time to design and manufacture this medical device.

The mechanical properties of the stent govern the decision process. This important property will be in charge of providing the correct longitudinal and radial behavior. The mechanical properties of the stents mainly depend on the material, geometry, and medical application of the stent:

$$\text{Mechanical properties} = f\,(\text{material, geometry, application}) \qquad (1)$$

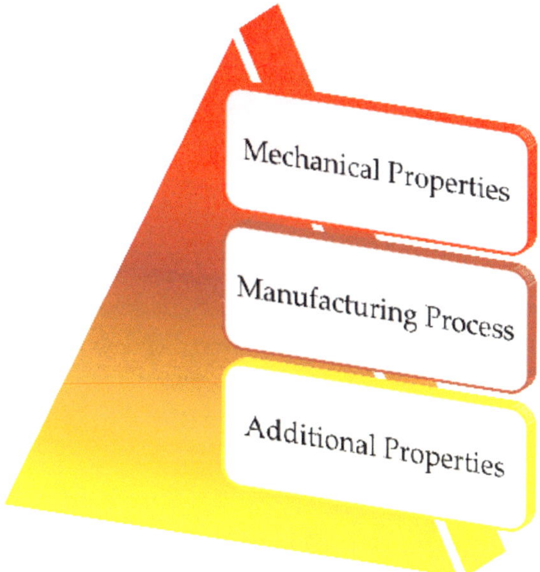

Figure 1. Pyramid of stent manufacturing process design.

Once we have decided the mechanical properties, we give way to the manufacturing process step. The manufacturing process mainly depends on the materials and stent type chosen:

$$\text{Manufacturing process} = f\,(\text{material, stent type}) \tag{2}$$

Finally, the additional properties step. Although it constitutes the final layer of the stent pyramid, additional properties cover a range of modifications to stent designs. This last step indirectly relates to the stent type and its medical application:

$$\text{Additional properties} = f\,(\text{stent type, application}) \tag{3}$$

The next sections present the main issues to consider in the abovementioned decision pyramid steps with special attention to the manufacturing process step.

3. Stent mechanical properties

Stent's mechanical properties are interrelated and sometimes contradictory, requiring careful compromise between geometrical and material aspects.

3.1. Geometrical aspects

Following the classification done by Stoeckel et al. in their manuscript "A survey of stent designs," stents can be classified into five categories [7].

3.1.1. Coil

Most common in nonvascular applications, the coil design allows for retrievability after implantation (**Figure 2a**). These designs are extremely flexible, but their strength is limited, and their low expansion ratio results in high-profile devices.

3.1.2. Helical spiral

These designs are generally promoted for their flexibility. With no or minimal internal connection points, they are very flexible but also lack longitudinal support. As such, they can be subject to elongation or compression during delivery and deployment and, consequently, irregular cell size. With internal connection points, some flexibility is sacrificed in exchange for longitudinal stability and additional control over cell size.

3.1.3. Woven

Woven designs are often used for self-expanding structures. While these designs offer excellent coverage, they typically shorten substantially during expansion. The radial strength of such a woven structure is also highly dependent on axial fixation of its ends.

3.1.4. Individual rings

These are commonly used to support grafts or similar prostheses. This design is not typically used as vascular stents by itself.

3.1.5. Sequential rings

This design is the most common in the market and includes two different categories: (I) closed cell, made of sequential ring construction wherein all internal inflection points of the structural members are connected (**Figure 2b**) and (II) open cells, a stent wherein some or all the internal inflection points of the structural member are not connected by bridging elements (**Figure 2c**).

3.2. Material aspects

Since the introduction of the first stainless steel devices, the materials used for stents have evolved and diversified rapidly. In the drive to obtain a share of what was becoming a vast and growing market, manufacturers invested heavily in research and development to gain continuous.

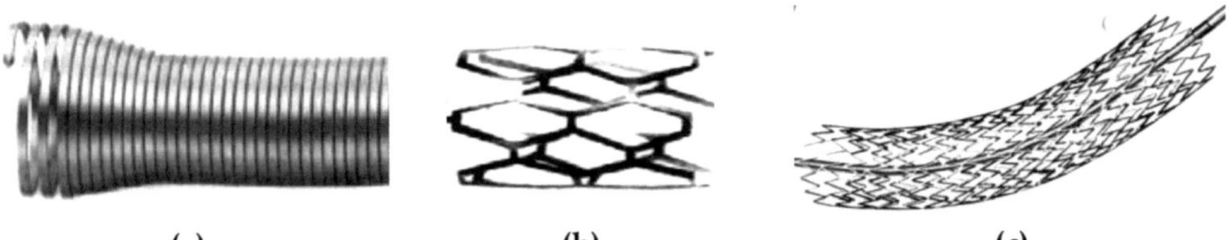

Figure 2. Designs: (a) coil EsophaCoil, (b) closed cell Palmaz-Schatz, and (c) open cell SMART.

The main materials currently used or which are being investigated are briefly presented in **Table 1**.

In the field of mechanical properties of stents, many authors have focused their investigations in the study of the effects of the geometry and the material that this medical device have. Due to the high cost of these medical devices, much of the works have been performed by finite element analysis (FEA).

In 2007, Kiousis et al. [8] proposed a methodology to identify optimal stents for specific clinical criteria. They presented a numerical study to understand the interaction between the stent and a patient-specific atherosclerotic human lesion of type V. Mortier et al. [9] compared three different second-generation drug-eluting stents (DES) using a parametric modeling approach, when being implanted in the curved main branch of a coronary bifurcation with the aim of providing better insights into the related changes of the mechanical environment. Hopkins et al. [10] carried out a study which provided insight into the critical factors governing coating delamination during stent deployment and offered a predictive framework that can be used to improve the design of coated stents. They concluded that delamination initiation is governed by coating thickness and stiffness, interface strength, and hinge curvature. Augsburger et al. [11] proposed an alternative strategy, which is based on the modeling of the device as porous medium. Results predicted by the porous medium approach compare well with the real stent

Type	Material	Description
Nondegradable	316 stainless steels (SS316)	It is also referred to as marine-grade stainless steel; is a chromium, nickel, and molybdenum alloy of steel that exhibits relatively good strength and corrosion resistance; and is a common choice for biomedical implants, such as stents
	Nitinol (NiTi)	Nitinol is a metal alloy of nickel and titanium, where the two elements are present in roughly equal atomic percentages. Nitinol alloys exhibit two closely related and unique properties—shape memory (SME) and superelasticity (SE)— perfect to self-expandable stents
Fully degradable	Magnesium (Mg)	Magnesium is the third most commonly used structural metal. Magnesium is used in super strong, lightweight materials and alloys. Magnesium alloys have been historically used by the magnesium tendency to corrode, creep at high temperature, and combust
	Poly-L-lactide acid (PLLA)	PLLA is a biodegradable thermoplastic aliphatic polyester derived from renewable resources, such as corn starch. Degradation is produced by hydrolysis of its ester linkages in physiological conditions
	Polycaprolactone (PCL)	PCL is a biodegradable polyester with a low melting point (60°C) and a glass transition of about −60°C. Degradation is produced by hydrolysis of its ester linkages in physiological conditions and has therefore received a great deal of attention

Table 1. Stent materials.

geometry model and allow predicting the main effects of the device on intra-aneurismal flow, facilitating thus the analysis. Hsiao et al. [12] proposed to apply the parametric design concept onto the stent design and integrate it with the developed FEA and CFD models to evaluate these key clinical attributes as a function of the stent design parameters. They concluded that the most critical parameter for the equivalent plastic strain and the expansion recoil was the crown radius. Grujicic et al. [13] investigated the fatigue-controlled service life of the self-expanding nitinol vascular stents. Praveen Kumar et al. [14] provided a simple, fast, and cost-effective tool to quantitatively determine the fatigue resistance of stent components. Their results showed that the stent model passed the fatigue test under the aforementioned loading conditions. Nowadays the main efforts are being done in simulating polymeric materials in order to understand the mechanical behavior of the new polymeric BRS [15, 16].

Stent materials have been investigated in-depth in the last decades. Understand how the manufacturing processes affect the material properties; develop new materials, analyses for new coating and its effect on the biological aspects, etc.; and have been the main research lines.

In 2010, Liu et al. [17] analyzed the inhibition of bacterial adherence on the surface of biliary stent made of 316L SS modified with chitosan. Bacterial infection plays an important role in the initiation of biliary sludge formation. Bacterial adherence and biofilm formation on the surface of a material have been considered as one of the main factors of stent re-occlusion in clinic. Results suggested that that chitosan could be applied to biliary stent in clinical setting because of its antimicrobial activities. In 2011, Man et al. [18] used a Nd:YAG laser to cut NiTi alloy employing air and argon environment, respectively. The corrosion resistance improved for samples treated in air.

In 2012, Ye [19] coated WE43 magnesium alloy with phytic acid (PA) by immersion. Authors aim to study the effect of PA's pH on the microstructure. Results showed that PA can enhance the corrosion resistance of WE43 magnesium especially when the pH value of the modified solution is 5 and the cytotoxicity of the PA-coated WE43 magnesium alloy is much better than that of the bare WE43 magnesium alloy. Moreover, all the hemolysis rates of the PA-coated WE43 Mg alloy were lower than 5%, indicating that the modified Mg alloy met the hemolysis standard of biomaterials. Therefore, PA coating is a good candidate to improve the biocompatibility of WE43 magnesium alloy.

The inclusion of BRS concepts was made that many author started to study bioresorbable materials. In the design of biodegradable stent, it is advantageous to consider materials that have received regulatory approval for other applications such as PLA. Other synthetic biodegradable polymers with regulatory approval have been attempted as stent materials, such as PCL, PGA, and P4HB. Regardless of polymer choice, the challenges associated with material formulation, polymerization process, material processing, and material property characterization remain similar. Most importantly, it is not only necessary to know the characteristics of the material at its initial non-degraded stage but also how do these evolve with degradation. The vast majority of studies of polymer degradation were performed without mechanical loading. The few studies that have included mechanical loading indicate that degradation is accelerated, depending on the specific type of loading. Wiggins et al. [20] found that the degradation rate of polyurethane increased with cyclic strain rate, whereas strain magnitude has essentially no effect. In a separate study, the same group demonstrated that polymer from the cyclic uniaxial strain region degraded at the same rate as unstressed and constant stress controls. In 2000, Tamai et al. [21] evaluated the feasibility, safety, and efficacy of the PLLA stent in humans. Fifteen patients electively underwent PLLA Igaki-Tamai stent implantation for coronary artery stenosis. The results were promising. Zilberman et al. [22] focused their studies on the mechanical properties of bioresorbable fibers. PLLA, PDS, and PGACL were studied in vitro. The three fibers combined a relatively high initial strength and modulus together with sufficient ductility. Venkatraman et al. [23] reported, for the first time, the development of a fully biodegradable polymeric stent that can self-expand at body temperatures. Ajili et al. [24] reported new self-expanding polymer made from polyurethane/polycaprolactone (PU/PCL). The results showed that the blend supported cell adhesion and proliferation, which indicated good biocompatibility. Their results suggested that this blend might be a potential material as a stent implant. Xue et al. [25] designed a biodegradable shape-memory block copolymer (PCTBV-25) for fast self-expandable stents. The stent made from PCTBV-25 film showed nearly complete self-expansion at 37°C within only 25 s, which is much better and faster than the best-known self-expandable stents. Vieira et al. [26] studied the evolution of mechanical properties during degradation based on experimental data. The decrease of tensile strength followed the same trend as the decrease of molecular weight. Weinandy et al. [27] designed a new viable stent structure (BioStent) to overcome in-stent restenosis. Despite the advances, many concerns still remain; one of the most important is the investigation on the cell proliferation of the material that helps to induce a rapid endothelialization.

4. Traditional stent manufacturing processes

Five technique has been used to manufacture stents: etching, micro-electro discharge machining, electroforming, die-casting, and, nowadays, laser cutting [28].

4.1. Etching

Etching method is based upon the photolithography process (**Figure 3a**). In this process, the desired mask pattern is first projected on the plain sheet coated with photoresist, which after exposure can be developed and etched for the desired pattern [29, 30].

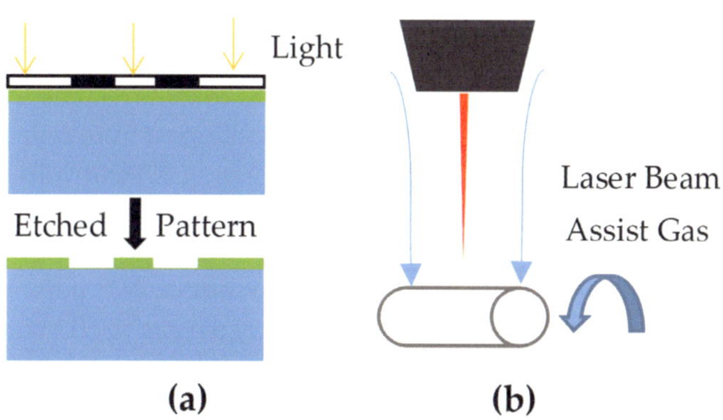

Figure 3. Stent manufacturing processes: (a) etching and (b) laser cutting.

4.2. Micro-EDM

In micro-EDM, the material removal takes place by electro-erosion due to electric discharge generated between closely spaced electrodes in the presence of a dielectric medium. The shape of the machined feature is the mirror image of electrode [31].

4.3. Electroforming

In this process, electroplating is performed on a mandrel in a given pattern. When the desired thickness has been reached, the mandrel is etched away from the electroformed stent, leaving a free standing structure, a fully functional stent [32, 33].

4.4. Die-casting

This is another technique in which the stent can also be formed by subjecting one or more. The metal may be cast directly in a stent-like form or cast into sheet or tubes from which the inventive stents are produced by using any of the method mentioned here.

4.5. Laser cutting

A high energy density laser beam is focused on workpiece surface; the thermal energy is absorbed which heats and transforms the workpiece volume into a molten, vaporized, or chemically changed state that can easily be removed by flow of high pressure assist gas jet [34, 35] (**Figure 3b**). Currently, this is the technology in the market.

Different types of lasers have been used in stent manufacture including CO_2 lasers, Nd:YAG lasers, fiber lasers, excimer lasers, and ultra-short pulse lasers. Fiber lasers have advantages compared to other laser technologies such as better beam quality, reliability, and process efficiency with lower acquisition cost and maintenance. Laser cutting is a thermal process which results in thermal damage such as heat-affected zone (HAZ), striation, recast layer, microcracks, tensile residual stress, and dross. To overcome the thermal damages, basically the following post-processing techniques are applied: pickling techniques, soft etching, annealing, and electropolishing. All these post-processing techniques raise the manufacture cost and could affect the mechanical properties of stents.

There are several works, which study how the process parameters affect the quality, trying to reduce the thermal problems and thus reduce the cost of the stent manufacturing process. Kathuria [36] described the precision fabrication of metallic stent from stainless steel by using short pulse Nd:YAG laser. They conclude that the processing of stent with desired taper and quality shall still be preferred by the short pulse and higher pulse repetition rate of the laser. Meng et al. [35] analyzed the cut parameters with a fiber laser system. They concluded that the high-quality coronary stent has been cut with the power of 7 W, pulse length of 0.15 ms, frequency of 1500 Hz, scanning speed of 8 mm/s, and oxygen gas at 0.3 MPa as assistance gas. Muhammad et al. [37] studied the capability of picosecond laser micromachining of nitinol and platinum-iridium alloy in improving the cut quality. Process parameters used in the process have achieved dross-free cut and minimum extent of HAZ. Scintilla and Tricarico [38] analyzed the influence of processing parameters and laser source type on cutting edge quality of AZ31 magnesium alloy sheet, and differences in cutting efficiency between fiber and CO_2 laser were studied. They investigate the effect of processing parameters in a laser cutting of 1 and 3.3-mm-thick sheets on the cutting quality. Their results showed that productivity, process efficiency, and cutting edge quality obtained using fiber lasers outperform CO_2 laser performances. Teixidor et al. [39] carried out an experimental study of fiber laser cutting of 316L stainless steel thin sheets. They analyzed the effect of laser parameters on the cutting quality for fixed nitrogen assistance gas. Besides that, they presented a mathematical model based on energy balance for the dross dimensions.

Notwithstanding, avoiding the thermal damages in laser processing is impossible by itself. Another alternative would be to solve it during the laser ablation process itself. This can be accomplished by laser machining under liquid. Laser processing in the presence of liquid has been studied for more than 40 years for various applications [40, 41]. Nevertheless underwater laser micromachining for tubes specifically for coronary stent applications received less attention. Work by Muhammad et al. [42] directed a water flow through the tubes during the fiber laser micromachining to reduce HAZ, as well as protecting the opposite surface of the tube. Yang et al. [43] reported underwater machining of deep cavities in alumina ceramic. They found that underwater machining has the capability of preventing crack initiation, reducing heat damage, and giving an insignificant recast layer. In other works, Muhammad and Li [44] studied the underwater femtosecond laser micromachining of thin nitinol tubes.

Despite the advances, the inclusion of the BRS concept should make us wonder about the applicability of the current laser-cutting manufacturing process for making BRS due to the new materials that have to be used, mostly polymers. There are several works about laser processing of biodegradable materials, both polymers and metals, trying to answer this question. Lootz et al. [45] analyzed the influence of laser-cutting process (CO_2 laser) in morphological and physicochemical properties of polyhydroxybutyrate. The result showed that cells preferred laser-machined areas. They concluded that not only were the material properties altered as a result of processing but also the biological response was affected. Grabow et al. [46] studied the effect of laser cutting on poly-L-lactide (PLLA). The results showed the dramatic influence of the plasticizer content and sterilization procedure on the mechanical properties of the material. Laser cutting had a lesser effect. Hence the effects of processing and sterilization must not be overlooked in the material selection and design phases of the development process leading to clinical use. Tiaw et al. [47] studied the effect of Nd:YAG laser on microdrilling and microcutting of thin PCL films. Melting and tearing of the thin polymer film were not much of an issue for the thin spin-cast film, but a slight extent of melting was observed in the thicker biaxial drawn film.

Baer et al. [48] described the fabrication of a laser-activated shape memory polymer (SMP) stent and demonstrated photothermal expansion of the stent in an in vitro artery model. In 2008, Davim et al. [49] realized some experimental studies on CO_2 laser cutting of polymeric materials. Their results showed that HAZ increases with the laser power and decreases with the cutting velocity. Yeong et al. [50] analyzed the effect of femtosecond laser micromachining on poly-E-caprolactone (PCL). Ortiz et al. [51] examined the picosecond laser ablation of PLLA as a function of laser fluence and degree of crystallinity. High-quality microgrooves were produced in amorphous PLLA, revealing the potential of ultra-fast laser processing technique. Demir et al. [52] demonstrated the feasibility of laser micro-cutting to produced magnesium BRS. By Q-switched fiber laser authors cut AZ31 magnesium alloy. The cutting process was followed by a subsequent chemical etching to clean the kerf and surface finish. Stepak et al. [53] presented the impact of the KrF excimer laser irradiation above the ablation threshold on physicochemical properties of biodegradable PLLA. It could be concluded that the usage of the 248 nm wavelength resulted in simultaneous ablation at the surface and photodegradation within the entire irradiated volume due to high penetration depth. Furthermore, the thermal activation originating from relaxation of excited chromophores to vibrationally excited ground states enhances the degradation process. Stepak et al. [54] fabricated a polymer-based biodegradable stent using a CO_2 laser. They noted that the high-temperature gradient during the process altered the properties of the material within the heat-affected zone (HAZ). Guerra et al. [55, 56] demonstrated the feasibility of fiber lasers of 1.8 μm of wavelength to cut polycaprolactone sheet with higher precisions. The process is barely affected by the material properties. Nowadays there are many authors that carry on this field trying to give an answer to the current problems. Nevertheless, the inclusion of BRS concept has motivated most of the researchers to move to new technologies. The next section presents the most promising manufacturing techniques under investigation nowadays for producing BRS.

5. Promising stent manufacturing processes

Despite the proved feasibility of laser cutting to produce BRS, both metallic and polymeric, there is a need to develop new technologies to produce these medical devices. In this context, additive manufacturing (AM) could be a more economical solution. AM refers to processes used to create a 3D object in which layers of material are formed under computer control. The use of this technology for stent manufacture is recent [57–64] and could be a really interesting method to produce stent. Mainly, there are four different AM technologies in the stent field.

5.1. Stereolithography (SL) processes

Stereolithography (SL) (**Figure 4b**) works by focusing an ultraviolet (UV) light or visible light onto a vat of photopolymerizable resin. It can differentiate three types of SL technologies, laser-based stereolithography (SLA), digital light processing (DLP), and very recently liquid crystal display (LCD).

5.2. Selective laser sintering (SLS)

Selective laser sintering (SLS) uses a laser as the power source to sinter powdered material (metals, polymers, etc.), aiming the laser automatically at points in space defined by a 3D model, binding the material together to create a solid structure.

5.3. Fused filament fabrication (FFF)

Also known as fused deposition modeling (FDM), here a hot thermoplastic is extruded from a temperature-controlled print head to produce fairly robust objects to a high degree of accuracy. The filament is melted into the extruder, which deposited the material onto a computer-controlled platform (**Figure 4a**). It can differentiate two FFF processes for stent manufacturing, (I) traditional Cartesian FFF or (II) novel tubular FFF.

5.4. Electrospinning (SE)

Electrospinning (SE) is a fiber production method which uses electric force to draw charged threads of polymer solution or polymer melts up to fiber diameter in the order of some hundred nanometers (**Figure 4c**). Traditionally, this technique has been used for coating permanent stents to produce DES.

In this new context, in the AM processes, some authors have focused their efforts to produce stents mainly focused on the new BRS. The novel use of polymeric materials joined with these new manufacturing methods opens a window to a novel concept, electrospun tubular bioabsorbable scaffold for stenting application. This new idea could reduce the problems derived from the current stents, such as its placements or rapid endothelialization.

Regarding the traditional BRS, the first document that presented a stent produced by AM was reported in 2015 when Park et al. [57] evaluated the properties of a 3D-printed BRS drug-coated stent in animals. Their results were promising in animals (20.7% restenosis). van Lith et al. [58] built a novel μCLIP setup capable of speed ranging from 2.5 to 100 μm s^{-1}. Employing a Cipher BMS design, they analyzed the effect of UV intensity, UV absorber, and wall thickness. Although results were promising, there are some limitations since the best-performing stent had a fabrication of 70 min. Misra et al. [61] performed an in silico analysis to optimize the stent design for printing and its prediction of sustainability under force exerted by the coronary artery or blood flow. Ware et al. [63] reported the process development in manufacturing high-resolution bioresorbable stents using the μCLIP system. They employed 26.5 min to manufacture a 2 cm stent. Cabrera et al. [62] manufactured a BRS stent employing a traditional 3D printer. Although the results were promising, the traditional 3D printer presents some limitations to manufacture tubular devices such as stent. Guerra et al. [59, 64] design and implement a novel 3D tubular printer to BRS manufacture, the first full research paper that applies 3D-printing process based on FFF to manufacture a BRS stent with nontraditional printer. Their approach presented a new and interesting method to produce stents based on polymers in less than 2 min (**Figure 5**).

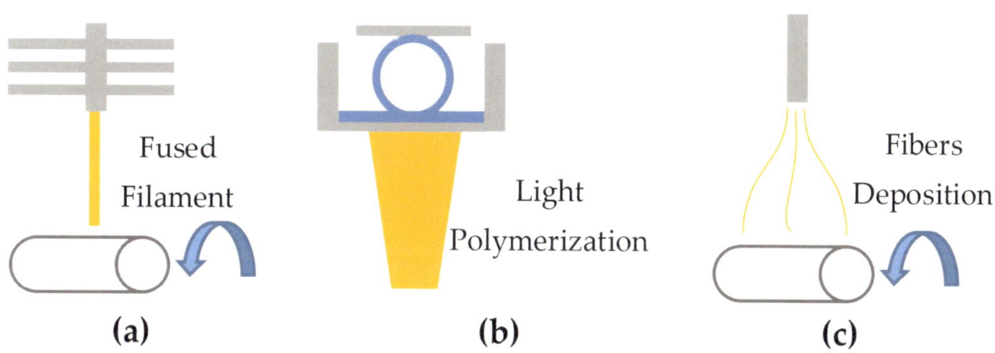

Figure 4. Promising manufacturing processes: (a) FFF, (b) SL, and (c) electrospinning.

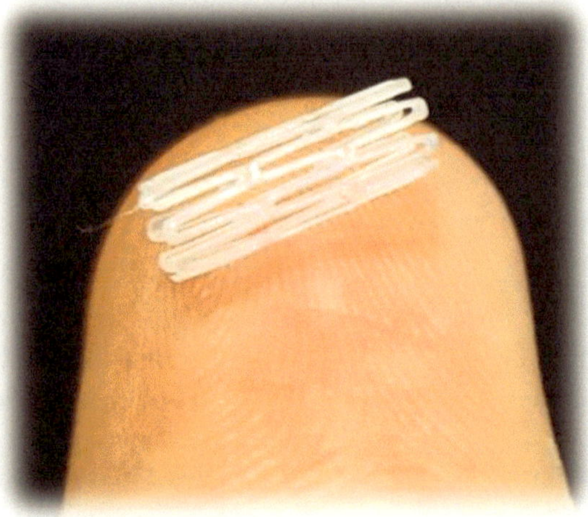

Figure 5. 3D-printed PCL stent [65].

Demir and Previtali [60] produced CoCr stent through SLM as an alternative method to the conventional manufacturing cycle. Results showed that SLM can be considered as a substitute operation to laser micro-cutting. Prototype stents with acceptable geometrical accuracy were achieved, and surface quality could be improved through electrochemical polishing. The chemical composition remained unvaried, with a marginal increase in the oxide content.

In recent studies, Guerra et al. [66] manufactured a PCL/PLA composite stent by FFF. They suggested that composite stents could improve the mechanical behavior of polymeric materials. Also, their results suggested that composite stents could improve the biological requirements, namely, high proliferation external surface, to help the endothelialization with low proliferation internal surface to avoid the adhesion and proliferation of the cell in charge of restenosis.

Regarding the novel electrospun tubular scaffolds (ETS) for stenting applications, some authors have been trying to produce them by electrospinning. Scaffold for stenting applications presents some advances as regards the traditional closed-cell stents. The longitudinal flexibility of scaffolds is higher than traditional stents, making their placement easy and reducing the risk during the stenting protocol. Also, scaffolds, produced by electrospinning, mimic the human tissue being able to increase the cell proliferation and helping a better and faster endothelialization of the vessel. However, scaffolds, due to their geometrical aspects can have worse radial behavior making it difficult for the vessel support. As a new idea, scaffold for stenting application has been barely studied. Bakola et al. [67] manufactured a drug-eluting bioabsorbable stent with PCL and PLA by electrospinning process. Authors focus their work in its application as coating to produce DES; nevertheless, results showed good morphology and topography. Nevertheless authors did not perform radial tests to check the feasibility of scaffold for stenting purposes. ETS present a new research field into the stent world. Further works that get into the manufacturing process and mechanical behavior of this new concept are completely necessary.

http://dx.doi.org/10.5772/intechopen.81668

AM process	Manufacturing issues			Final stent properties		
	Costs	Speeds	Precisions	Radial	Longitudinal	Biological
SL	poor	poor	good	poor	poor	poor
SLS	poor	poor	good	poor	poor	poor
Traditional FFF	good	good	medium	poor	poor	poor
Tubular FFF	good	good	medium	good	medium	medium
ES	good	medium	poor	poor	good	good

■ (red), poor property; ■ (green), good property; ■ (blue), medium property

Table 2. Additive manufacturing (AM) process advantages and disadvantages.

AM processes have proved their effectiveness, and clearly they present a novel method to produce stents that could replace the current laser-cutting process. Depending on the AM process use, the manufacturer will have some advantages and disadvantages. **Table 2** summarized some on them.

Despite the few works about AM of stents, results have proved that these techniques could be promising. Further studies with new materials and technologies become crucial to understand the effect the process parameters has on stent properties and enclose the best material and process.

6. Additional properties

Although it constitutes the final layer of the stent manufacturing pyramid, additional properties cover a range of modifications to stent designs that sometimes become crucial. This section presents briefly the most common additional properties that are added to the stents.

6.1. Radiopacity markers

Stents made from stainless steel, nitinol, or polymers are sometimes hard to see fluoroscopically, particularly if they are small and/or have thin and narrow struts. To improve X-ray visibility, markers are often attached to the stents. These additions are typically made from gold, platinum, or tantalum and can be sleeves crimped around a strut [7].

6.2. Drug release

It is the main additional property usually added to stents in the current clinic practice. The main stent currently used in clinic is DES. There are a variety of coating techniques to incorporate drugs to the stent [68]. **Table 3** briefly presents the most common techniques.

Multiple variables can be adjusted to optimize drug release for cardiovascular stent applications, including biocompatible polymers and antirestenotic drugs. While the presence of a

Technique	Brief description
Dip coating	Coating by submerging the stent in a solution of drug and/or polymer in a solvent. The stent is then left to dry, allowing for evaporation, in the air/oven. In this technique the drug/polymer can vary their concentration and/or their homogeneity
Electro-treated coating	The drug/polymer particles are suspended in a liquid medium migrate under the influence of an electric field and are deposited onto an electrode (stent)
Plasma-treated coating	Plasma coating (plasma activation) is a method of surface modification which improves surface adhesion properties. Plasma produce a reduction of metal oxides, surface cleaning from organic contaminants, and modification of the topography
Spray coating	These techniques use apparatuses that spray polymer and drug solutions (using various solvents) onto a stent, enabling consistent deposit of a uniform drug release layer(s) onto the stent surface

Table 3. Most common coating techniques in stent manufacturing industry.

polymer coating on a DES is not required, the process to choose one can be difficult because it has been previously shown that most polymers listed as biocompatible and used in medicine can cause vascular inflammation.

7. Summary

Stents have been the center of many research lines in the last decades. The challenges associated with this medical device are numerous: geometry, material, manufacturing process, biocompatibility, etc. Finite element analysis (FEA) studies have been trying to understand the role of the different geometrical and material aspects in the mechanical behavior of stents. Material studies have been developing new material that accomplishes with the stent requirements in terms of mechanical and medical properties, both in the permanent field and in the biodegradable field. Finally, in the manufacturing research field, authors have been focused in improving the process by analyzing the parameters to obtain a stent with the higher precision and the minimal costs. In this research line, there are noteworthy lines: laser micro-cutting and, more recently, additive manufacturing. Additive manufacturing studies are showing their huge potential in the field of polymeric BRS.

There is a need to develop techniques for evaluating the ability of biodegradable stents to provide not only acute support but also reliable structural integrity for an appropriate period of time. In all these properties, the material and manufacturing process plays an important role. To achieve this, the previously mentioned research fields should be converged. The FEA field is developing new geometries with bioabsorbable polymer such as polycaprolactone that accomplishes with the stent mechanical requirements. The material field is developing new materials that accomplish the strict stent requirements. In the case of metallic alloys, develop material degraded with an appropriate rate. In the case of polymers, develop material accomplish with the mechanical and manufacturing properties of metallic ones. Lastly, the manufacturing process field should work to increase the knowledge about the process parameters to obtain a more accurate result in the case of tubular FFF process and faster production in the case of SL processes that nowadays are presented as the most promising technique under investigation. Also, further works about ETS are necessary. ETS present a new research field into the stent world that could solve some current medical problems. Finally, the sterilization process should be noted. This last but mandatory manufacturing step could be critical for the final properties of stents. As Grabow et al. [46], or more recently Guerra et al. [65], have demonstrated, sterilization processes can change the final properties. Further works that get into the effect the sterilization processes has on stent properties are completely necessary.

Acknowledgements

Authors acknowledge the financial support from the Ministry of Economy and Competitiveness (MINECO, DPI2016-77156-R), the University of Girona (UDG, MPCUdG2016/036), and the Catalan government (2017SGR00385).

Conflict of interest

The authors declare no conflict of interest.

Author details

Antonio J. Guerra and Joaquim Ciurana*

*Address all correspondence to: quim.ciurana@udg.edu

Department of Mechanical Engineering and Civil Construction, Universitat de Girona, Girona, Spain

References

[1] Grüntzig A. Transluminal dilatation of coronary artery stenosis. Lancet. 1978;**1**(C):263. Available from: http://scholar.google.com/scholar?hl=en&btnG=Search&q=intitle:Transluminal+dilatation+of+coronary+artery+stenosis#0

[2] Serruys PW, de Jaegere P, Kiemeneij F, Macaya C, Rutsch W, Heyndrickx G, et al. A comparison of balloon-expandable-stent implantation with balloon angioplasty in patients with coronary artery disease. The New England Journal of Medicine. 1994;**331**:489-495

[3] Schwartz RS, Topol EJ, Serruys PW, Sangiorgi G, Holmes DRJ. Artery size, neointima, and remodeling: Time for some standards. Journal of the American College of Cardiology. 1998;**32**(7):2087-2094

[4] Waksman R. Update on bioabsorbable stents: From bench to clinical. Journal of Interventional Cardiology. 2006;**19**(5):414-421

[5] Rabionet M, Yeste M, Puig T, Ciurana J. Electrospinning PCL scaffolds manufacture for three-dimensional breast cancer cell culture. Polymers (Basel). 2017;**9**(8):328

[6] Medipoint. Coronary Stents—Global Analysis and Market Forecasts. 2014;34. Available from: https://www.marketresearch.com/product/sample-8538829.pdf

[7] Stoeckel D, Bonsignore C, Duda S. A Survey of stent design. Cell. 2002;**11**(4):137-147

[8] Kiousis DE, Gasser TC, Holzapfel GA. A numerical model to study the interaction of vascular stents with human atherosclerotic lesions. Annals of Biomedical Engineering. 2007;**35**(11):1857-1869

[9] Mortier P, Holzapfel GA, De Beule M, Van Loo D, Taeymans Y, Segers P, et al. A novel simulation strategy for stent insertion and deployment in curved coronary bifurcations: Comparison of three drug-eluting stents. Annals of Biomedical Engineering. 2010;**38**(1):88-99

[10] Hopkins CG, McHugh PE, McGarry JP. Computational investigation of the delamination of polymer coatings during stent deployment. Annals of Biomedical Engineering. 2010;**38**(7):2263-2273

[11] Augsburger L, Reymond P, Rufenacht DA, Stergiopulos N. Intracranial stents being modeled as a porous medium: Flow simulation in stented cerebral aneurysms. Annals of Biomedical Engineering. 2011;**39**(2):850-863

[12] Hsiao HM, Chiu YH, Lee KH, Lin CH. Computational modeling of effects of intravascular stent design on key mechanical and hemodynamic behavior. Computer-Aided Design. 2012;**44**(8):757-765. DOI: 10.1016/j. cad.2012.03.009

[13] Grujicic M, Pandurangan B, Arakere A, Snipes JS. Fatigue-life computational analysis for the self-expanding endovascular nitinol stents. Journal of Materials Engineering and Performance. 2012;**21**(11):2218-2230

[14] Praveen Kumar G, Cui F, Danpinid A, Su B, Hon JKF, Leo HL. Design and finite element-based fatigue prediction of a new self-expandable percutaneous mitral valve stent. Computer-Aided Design. 2013;**45**(10):1153-1158. DOI: 10.1016/j. cad.2013.05.003

[15] Welch TR, Eberhart RC, Banerjee S, Chuong C-J. Mechanical interaction of an expanding coiled stent with a plaque-containing arterial wall: A finite element analysis. Cardiovascular Engineering and Technology. 2016;**7**(1):58-68

[16] Bobel AC, Petisco S, Sarasua JR, Wang W, McHugh PE. Computational bench testing to evaluate the short-term mechanical performance of a polymeric stent. Cardiovascular Engineering and Technology. 2015;**6**(4):519-532

[17] Liu H, Huang N, Leng Y, Yu H, Le L, Li K. Inhibition of bacterial adherence on the surface of biliary stent materials modified with chitosan. Journal Wuhan University of Technology Materials Science Edition. 2010;**25**(5):795-798

[18] Man HC, Cui ZD, Yue TM. Corrosion properties of laser surface melted NiTi shape memory alloy. Scripta Materialia. 2001;**45**(12):1447-1453

[19] Ye CH, Zheng YF, Wang SQ, Xi TF, Li YD. In vitro corrosion and biocompatibility study of phytic acid modified WE43 magnesium alloy. Applied Surface Science. 2012;**258**(8): 3420-3427

[20] Wiggins MJ, Anderson JM, Hiltner A. Effect of strain and strain rate on fatigue-accelerated biodegradation of polyurethane. Journal of Biomedical Materials Research. Part A. 2003;**66**(3):463-475

[21] Tamai H, Igaki K, Kyo E, Kosuga K, Kawashima A, Matsui S, et al. Initial and 6-month results of biodegradable poly-l-lactic acid coronary stents in humans. Circulation. 2000; **102**(4):399-404. Available from: http://circ.ahajournals.org/content/102/4/399.abstract

[22] Zilberman M, Nelson KD, Eberhart RC. Mechanical properties and in vitro degradation of bioresorbable fibers and expandable fiber-based stents. Journal of Biomedical Materials Research Part B: Applied Biomaterials. 2005;**74**(2):792-799

[23] Venkatraman SS, Tan LP, Joso JFD, Boey YCF, Wang X. Biodegradable stents with elastic memory. Biomaterials. 2006;**27**(8):1573-1578

[24] Ajili SH, Ebrahimi NG, Soleimani M. Polyurethane/polycaprolactane blend with shape memory effect as a proposed material for cardiovascular implants. Acta Biomaterialia. 2009;**5**(5):1519-1530. DOI: 10.1016/j.actbio.2008.12.014

[25] Xue L, Dai S, Li Z. Biodegradable shape-memory block co-polymers for fast self-expandable stents. Biomaterials. 2010;**31**(32):8132-8140. DOI: 10.1016/j.biomaterials.2010.07.043

[26] Vieira AC, Vieira JC, Ferra JM, Magalhães FD, Guedes RM, Marques AT. Mechanical study of PLA-PCL fibers during in vitro degradation. Journal of the Mechanical Behavior of Biomedical Materials. 2011;**4**(3):451-460. DOI: 10.1016/j.jmbbm.2010.12.006

[27] Weinandy S, Rongen L, Schreiber F, Cornelissen C, Flanagan TC, Mahnken A, et al. The BioStent: Novel concept for a viable stent structure. Tissue Engineering. Part A. 2012; **18**(17-18):1818-1826

[28] Kathuria YP. The potential of biocompatible metallic stents and preventing restenosis. Materials Science and Engineering A. 2006;**417**(1-2):40-48

[29] Fuchsberger K, Binder K, Burkhardt C, Freudigmann C, Herrmann M, Stelzle M. Electrochemical etching of micro-pores in medical grade cobalt–chromium alloy as reservoirs for drug eluting stents. Journal of Materials Science. Materials in Medicine. 2016;**27**(3):1-9

[30] Galvin E, Morshed MM, Cummins C, Daniels S, Lally C, MacDonald B. Surface modification of absorbable magnesium stents by reactive ion etching. Plasma Chemistry and Plasma Processing. 2013;**33**(6):1137-1152

[31] Takahata K, Gianchandani YB. Coronary artery stents microfabricated from planar metal foil: Design, fabrication, and mechanical testing. In: Proceedings of the IEEE Micro Electro Mechanical Systems (MEMS). 2003. pp. 462-465

[32] Moravej M, Purnama A, Fiset M, Couet J, Mantovani D. Electroformed pure iron as a new biomaterial for degradable stents: In vitro degradation and preliminary cell viability studies. Acta Biomaterialia. 2010;**6**(5):1843-1851

[33] Wang WQ, Wang J, Qi M. Microstructure and in vitro biodegradable properties of Fe-Zn alloys prepared by electroforming. Advanced Materials Research. 2014;**1033-1034**: 1200-1206

[34] Meng H, Liao J, Zhou Y, Zhang Q. Laser micro-processing of cardiovascular stent with fiber laser cutting system. Optics and Laser Technology. 2009;**41**(3):300-302

[35] Meng H-Y, Liao J-H, Guan B-G, Zhang Q-M, Zhou Y-H. Fiber laser cutting technology on coronary artery stent. Chinese Journal of Lasers. 2007;**34**(5):733-736

[36] Kathuria YP. Laser microprocessing of metallic stent for medical therapy. Journal of Materials Processing Technology. 2005;**170**(3):545-550

[37] Muhammad N, Whitehead D, Boor A, Oppenlander W, Liu Z, Li L. Picosecond laser micromachining of nitinol and platinum-iridium alloy for coronary stent applications. Applied Physics A: Materials Science & Processing. 2012;**106**(3):607-617

[38] Scintilla LD, Tricarico L. Experimental investigation on fiber and CO_2 inert gas fusion cutting of AZ31 magnesium alloy sheets. Optics & Laser Technology. 2013;**46**:42-52. DOI: 10.1016/j.optlastec.2012.04.026

[39] Teixidor D, Ciurana J, Rodriguez CA. Dross formation and process parameters analysis of fibre laser cutting of stainless steel thin sheets. International Journal of Advanced Manufacturing Technology. 2014;**71**(9-12):1611-1621. DOI: 10.1007/s00170-013-5599-0

[40] Kruusing A. Underwater and water-assisted laser processing: Part 1—General features, steam cleaning and shock processing. Optics and Lasers in Engineering. 2004;**41**:307-327

[41] Kruusing A. Underwater and water-assisted laser processing: Part 2—Etching, cutting and rarely used methods. Optics and Lasers in Engineering. 2004;**41**(2):329-352

[42] Muhammad N, Whitehead D, Boor A, Li L. Comparison of dry and wet fibre laser profile cutting of thin 316L stainless steel tubes for medical device applications. Journal of Materials Processing Technology. 2010;**210**(15):2261-2267

[43] Yang J, Cui F, Lee IS. Surface modifications of magnesium alloys for biomedical applications. Annals of Biomedical Engineering. 2011;**39**(7):1857-1871

[44] Muhammad N, Li L. Underwater femtosecond laser micromachining of thin nitinol tubes for medical coronary stent manufacture. Applied Physics A: Materials Science & Processing. 2012;**107**(4):849-861

[45] Lootz D, Behrend D, Kramer S, Freier T, Haubold A, Benkießer G, et al. Laser cutting: Influence on morphological and physicochemical properties of polyhydroxybutyrate. Biomaterials. 2001;**22**(18):2447-2452

[46] Grabow N, Schlun M, Sternberg K, Hakansson N, Kramer S, Schmitz K-P. Mechanical properties of laser cut poly(L-lactide) micro-specimens: Implications for stent design, manufacture, and sterilization. Journal of Biomechanical Engineering. 2005;**127**(February):25-31

[47] Tiaw KS, Hong MH, Teoh SH. Precision laser micro-processing of polymers. Journal of Alloys and Compounds. 2008;**449**(1-2):228-231

[48] Baer GM, Small W, Wilson TS, Benett WJ, Matthews DL, Hartman J, et al. Fabrication and in vitro deployment of a laser-activated shape memory polymer vascular stent. Biomedical Engineering Online. 2007;**6**:43

[49] Davim JP, Barricas N, Conceição M, Oliveira C. Some experimental studies on CO_2 laser cutting quality of polymeric materials. Journal of Materials Processing Technology. 2008; **198**(1-3):99-104

[50] Yeong WY, Lim KP, Ka Lai Ng G, Tan LP, Yin Chiang Boey F, Venkatraman SS. Annealing of biodegradable polymer induced by femtosecond laser micromachining. Advanced Engineering Materials. 2010;**12**(4):89-93

[51] Ortiz R, Quintana I, Etxarri J, Lejardi A, Sarasua JR. Picosecond laser ablation of poly-L-lactide: Effect of crystallinity on the material response. Journal of Applied Physics. 2011;**110**(9):1-10

[52] Demir AG, Previtali B, Biffi CA. Fibre laser cutting and chemical etching of AZ31 for manufacturing biodegradable stents. Advances in Materials Science and Engineering. 2013;**2013**:1-11

[53] Stepak BD, Antończak AJ, Szustakiewicz K, Koziol PE, Abramski KM. Degradation of poly(l-lactide) under KrF excimer laser treatment. Polymer Degradation and Stability. 2014;**110**:156-164

[54] Stepak B, Antończak AJ, Bartkowiak-Jowsa M, Filipiak J, Pezowicz C, Abramski KM. Fabrication of a polymer-based biodegradable stent using a CO_2 laser. Archives of Civil and Mechanical Engineering. 2014;**14**(2):317-326

[55] Guerra AJ, Farjas J, Ciurana J. Fibre laser cutting of polycaprolactone sheet for stents manufacturing : A feasibility study. Optics & Laser Technology. 2017;**95**:113-123. DOI: 10.1016/j.optlastec.2017.03.048

[56] Guerra AJ, Ciurana J. Effect of fibre laser process on in-vitro degradation rate of a polycaprolactone stent a novel degradation study method. Polymer Degradation and Stability. 2017;**142**:42-49. Available from: http://linkinghub.elsevier.com/retrieve/pii/S0141391017301520

[57] Park SA, Lee SJ, Lim KS, Bae IH, Lee JH, Kim WD, et al. In vivo evaluation and characterization of a bio-absorbable drug-coated stent fabricated using a 3D-printing system. Materials Letters. 2015;**141**:355-358. DOI: 10.1016/j.matlet.2014.11.119

[58] van Lith R, Baker E, Ware H, Yang J, Farsheed AC, Sun C, et al. 3D-printing strong high-resolution antioxidant bioresorbable vascular stents. Advanced Materials Technologies. 2016;**1**(9):1600138. DOI: 10.1002/admt.201600138

[59] Guerra A, Roca A, de Ciurana J. A novel 3D additive manufacturing machine to biodegradable stents. Procedia Manufacturing. 2017;**13**:718-723. DOI: 10.1016/j.promfg.2017.09.118

[60] Demir AG, Previtali B. Additive manufacturing of cardiovascular CoCr stents by selective laser melting. Materials & Design. 2017;**119**:338-350. DOI: 10.1016/j.matdes.2017.01.091

[61] Misra SK, Ostadhossein F, Babu R, Kus J, Tankasala D, Sutrisno A, et al. 3D-printed multi-drug-eluting stent from graphene-nanoplatelet-doped biodegradable polymer composite. Advanced Healthcare Materials. 2017;**6**(11):1-14

[62] Cabrera MS, Sanders B, Goor OJGM, Driessen-Mol A, Oomens CW, Baaijens FPT. Computationally designed 3D printed self-expandable polymer stents with biodegradation capacity for minimally invasive heart valve implantation: A proof-of-concept study. 3D Printing and Additive Manufacturing. 2017;**4**(1):19-29. DOI: 10.1089/3dp.2016.0052

[63] Ware HOT, Farsheed AC, van Lith R, Baker E, Ameer G, Sun C. Process development for high-resolution 3D-printing of bioresorbable vascular stents. Biomedical Engineering Mechanical Engineering. 2017;**10115**:101150N. Available from: http://proceedings.spiedigitallibrary.org/proceeding.aspx?doi=10.1117/12.2252856

[64] Guerra A, Ciurana J. 3D-printed bioabsordable polycaprolactone stent: The effect of process parameters on its physical features. Materials & Design. 2018;**137**:430-437. Available from: http://www.sciencedirect.com/science/article/pii/S0264127517309723

[65] Guerra AJ, Cano P, Rabionet M, Puig T. Effects of different sterilization processes on the properties of a novel 3D-printed polycaprolactone stent. Polymers for Advanced Technologies. August 2018;**29**(8):2327-2335

[66] Guerra A, Cano P, Rabionet M, Puig T, Ciurana J. 3D-printed PCL/PLA composite stents: Towards a new solution to cardiovascular problems. Materials (Basel). 2018;**11**(9):1679. Available from: http://www.mdpi.com/1996-1944/11/9/1679

[67] Bakola V, Karagkiozaki V, Pappa F, Tsiapla AR, Pavlidou E, Moutsios I, et al. Drug delivery nanosystems for cardiovascular stents. Materials Today: Proceedings. 2017;**4**(7): 6869-6879. DOI: 10.1016/j.matpr.2017.07.016

[68] Livingston M, Tan A. Coating techniques and release kinetics of drug-eluting stents. Journal of Medical Devices. 2015;**10**(1):010801. Available from: http://medicaldevices.asmedigitalcollection.asme.org/article.aspx?doi=10.1115/1.4031718

Chapter 5

Dedicated Bifurcation Stents

Ivo Petrov, Iveta Tasheva, Jivka Stoykova,
Liubomir Dosev, Zoran Stankov and Petar Polomski

Additional information is available at the end of the chapter

http://dx.doi.org/10.5772/intechopen.82573

Abstract

Bifurcations still remain one of the most challenging lesions to be treated in the modern PCI era. They are associated with lower procedural success rates, higher rates of periprocedural complications, and complicated long-term outcomes. Their incidence is assessed to be approximately 15–20%. There is still debate on how should they be treated—one-stent versus two-stent techniques, whether there is a need for obligatory proximal optimization or kissing balloons. Multiple clinical trials have tested different PCI strategies. We will cover theoretical basics of treating bifurcations and describe different types of dedicated bifurcation stents—Nile PAX, Nile SIR, BiOSS Expert, BiOSS LIM, Stentys, Tryton, and Axxess Plus. We will discuss the data from studies comparing these bifurcation devices and will show our own experience and results working with these devices. There will be a discussion, tips, and tricks treating bifurcation lesions with dedicated devices—most common pitfalls and how to deal with them.

Keywords: bifurcation, left main, new devices

1. Introduction

Bifurcations still remain one of the most challenging lesions to be treated in the modern PCI era. They are associated with lower procedural success rates, higher rates of periprocedural complications, and complicated long-term outcomes. Their incidence is assessed to be approximately 15–20%. There is still debate on how should they be treated—one-stent versus two-stent techniques, whether there is a need for obligatory proximal optimization or kissing balloons. Multiple clinical trials have tested different PCI strategies.

The conventional stents are not designed for bifurcations as there is huge variation in vessel anatomy, mostly discrepancy in proximal and distal diameter of the treated vessel and a need for free access in the side branch. One major problem in bifurcation PCI is the high rate of SB ostium restenosis. There are also several procedural difficulties such as maintaining access to the side branch, irregular overlapping, and uneven distribution of struts at the carina. The final result and long-term success rates are highly variable and are operator dependent.

Closure of side branch bigger than 1 mm often is associated with 14% incidence of periprocedural myocardial infarction [1].

The dedicated bifurcation stents are produced to tackle most of these problems.

Dedicated bifurcation stents give hope for technically straightforward and fast success rate; they aim to protect the SB and allow permanent SB access as well as optimal MB and SB scaffolding and coverage. They also tend to limit multiple layering of stent struts, limit gaps in support, and prevent restenosis reducing SB risk, optimizing immediate and long-term outcomes.

2. Anatomy, physiology, and conventional stent treatment

Coronary bifurcation lesions should be viewed as three major parts—proximal main branch, distal main branch, and a side branch. Significant side branch is defined on the subjective judgment of the operator, which warrants its diameter, length, size of myocardial mass supplied, its viability, and left ventricular function.

Treating a bifurcation comes with the risk of losing SB patency; thus, the operator should thoroughly review the plaque burden at the carina, its angle, and diameter of MB and SB.

The MADS classification presents various techniques used in bifurcation stenting. There is one-stent (provisional) or two-stent strategy. Provisional stent strategy is done in majority of cases; it is recommended by the European Bifurcation Club as KISSS principle (Keep It Simple, Swift and Safe). At first, the MV is stented, the stent diameter is 1:1 according to distal MB diameter, and then operator should perform POT (proximal optimization technique) and eventually kissing balloon inflation. POT presents short oversized balloon dilation at proximal part of the stent (from proximal edge of the stent to proximal carina edge). This technique apposes stent struts to the proximal MV and enhances scaffolding at the SB ostium. After this, if operator decides based on SB ostium stenosis and flow, kissing balloon inflation could be done. Kissing inflation involves rewiring of the SB from the distal strut at SB ostium, and getting a balloon through the stent struts could be the most challenging part of bifurcation treatment. After rewiring, two NC balloons are simultaneously inflated in MB and SB.

After POT and kissing, if there is a need for SB stenting because of low flow or SB dissection, there are basically few strategies—T stenting, TAP (T stenting and protrusion), culotte, and crush techniques. In all two-stent techniques, kissing balloon dilation is mandatory to achieve full stent expansion at both ostia; sometimes, final POT should be considered.

T-stenting strategy is chosen when there is scaffolding at the SB ostium from the POT and when SB angulation is nearly 90°. If SB is not covered by POT technique and the angle is acute, crush (minicrush), culotte, and TAP should be considered as they all cover SB ostium with struts. In crush (minicrush), the stent in SB is placed overlapping the MB and is crushed with oversized balloon; finally, kissing balloons should be inflated. In culotte, SB stent also covers some of the MB and this part in MB is overexpanded with POT, leaving double strut layer at the proximal MB; final kissing is a must. More modern minicrush and miniculotte use shorter stent overlapping, thus decreasing strut burden. In Tap, the SB stent is left to protrude a bit proximal to carina, while leaving a balloon in MB for simultaneous kissing, thus making a neostrut carina.

Sometimes, if there is a large and diseased SB prone to ischemia and deterioration in LV function (mostly in left main), a two-stent strategy is chosen instead of provisional stent. It is operator's decision which part MB or SB to be stented first and which of two-stent strategies to choose.

Bioresorbable stents, besides their potential advantage to dissolve with time, have a lot of limitations—they are thicker (some techniques require multiple struts layers and you cannot always go with provisional one-stent strategy) and have limited expansion property and increased rates of thrombosis. Absorb BRS (Abbott Vascular USA) is already taken down from market. DESolve BRS (Elixir Medical USA) and Magmaris (BIOTRONIK Germany) could be a choice, but still there are a few data.

There are several devices dedicated to bifurcation treatment.

3. Tryton and Tryton SHORT stents

One of them is the dedicated bifurcational stents, Tryton and Tryton SHORT stents.

The delivery system of the stent is based on rapid-exchange catheter with single-wire tracking (no risk of wire wrap or bias); there is no need for rotational orientation. The stent has low profile and is 5-Fr guide compatible with two central markers delineating central transition zone used to precisely position the stent (**Figures 1–3**).

The deployment sequence of the stent consists of wiring the side branch and predilatation. Then, Tryton is positioned and is deployed from main branch to the side branch, after which the main branch is wired and a DES is positioned 1 mm proximal to the Tryton proximal edge. After deploying the stent in the main branch, rewiring of side branch and kissing is performed.

There are several drawbacks of Tryton system. It is a bare metal stent with consistently <5% TLR in all clinical studies in over 1.800 pts. It requires adequate proximal landing zone and accurate positioning, but the learning curve is short. It is not indicated for <2.25 mm vessels and is tied to two-stent strategy as intention to treat.

There are several randomized studies as far as this stent is concerned.

TRYTON randomized 704 patients with bifurcation coronary lesions at 58 centers (30 from Europe and 28 from the United States). At 9 months, TVF was 4.6% higher in the bifurcation stent group compared with the provisional group ($p = 0.11$). TVF was mainly presented by higher rates of periprocedural myocardial infarction rate (13.6 vs. 10.1%). The SB in-segment diameter stenosis was lower in the bifurcation stent group compared with the provisional group (31.6 vs. 38.6%), with no difference in binary restenosis rates (diameter stenosis ≥50%) at 9 months follow-up (22.6 vs. 26.8%) [2].

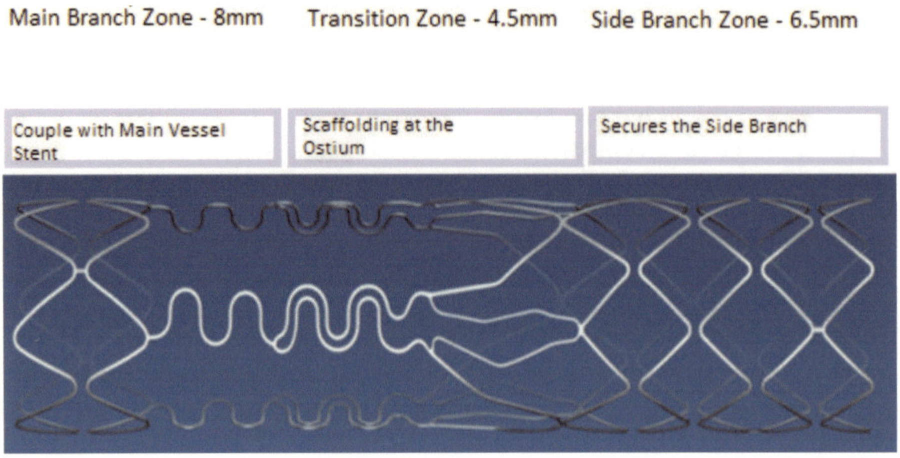

Figure 1. Tryton structure. It is cobalt-chromium balloon expandable stent. The strut thickness is 85 mkm and the total length of the stent is 19 mm. The transition zone can flare and rotate in order to accommodate the atomic variations of the side branch ostium and scaffolds like a main vessel stent at the ostium.

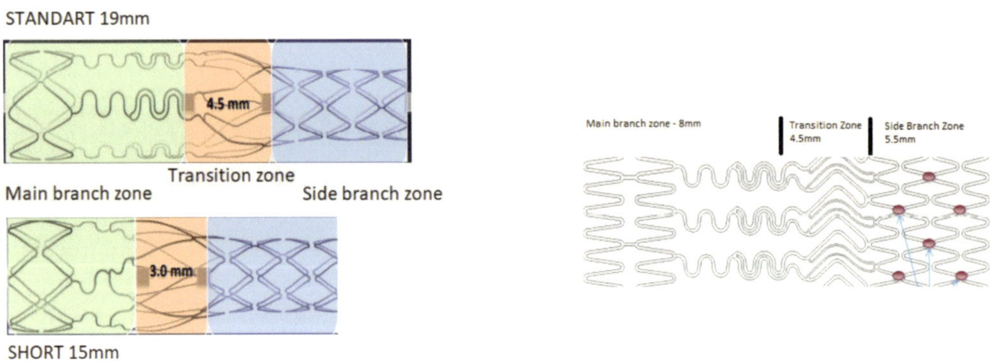

Figure 2. Tryton and Tryton SHORT stents. The proximal part of the main branch zone was designed to accommodate larger expansion, and the side branch zone is with additional links in order to increase radial force of the stent. The SHORT stent has 3 mm shorter landing zone, and the position of central markers is optimized for large vessels and has improved delivery system.

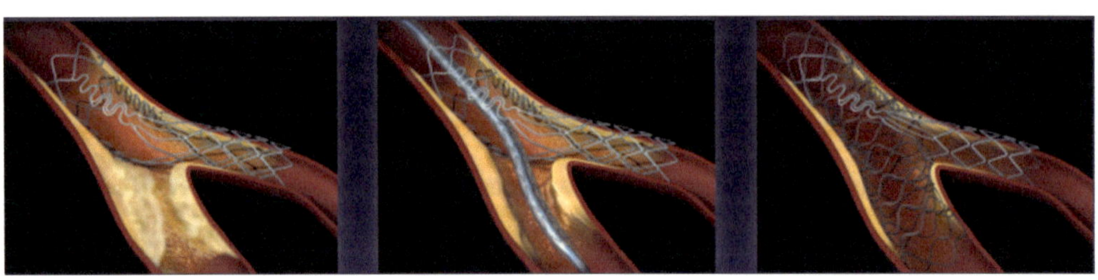

Figure 3. Tryton deployment scheme. The stent is positioned and deployed after predilatation (secures and protects side branch). The next pictures show treatment of main vessel with approved DES through main vessel portion of Tryton. The final step is kissing balloon postdilatation to ensure complete lesion and ostium coverage. Source: Genereux [3].

http://dx.doi.org/10.5772/intechopen.82573

After TRYTON study, a subanalysis of it examines the benefit of the Tryton compared with provisional stenting in treatment of complex bifurcation lesions involving large SB. Among the 704 patients enrolled in the TRYTON trial, 289 patients (143 provisional and 146 Tryton stent)

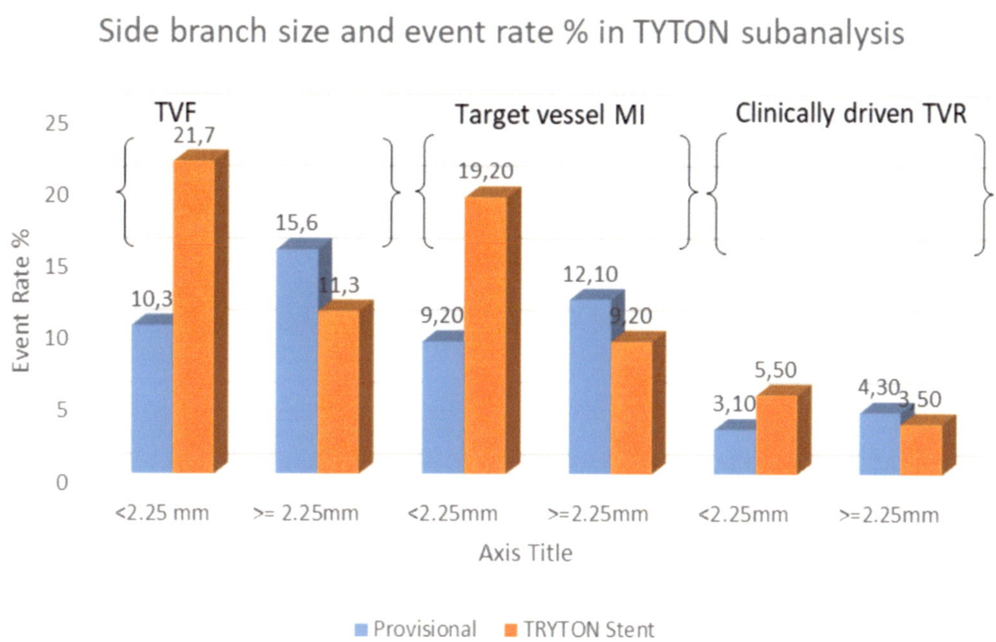

Figure 4. TRYTON subanalysis results.

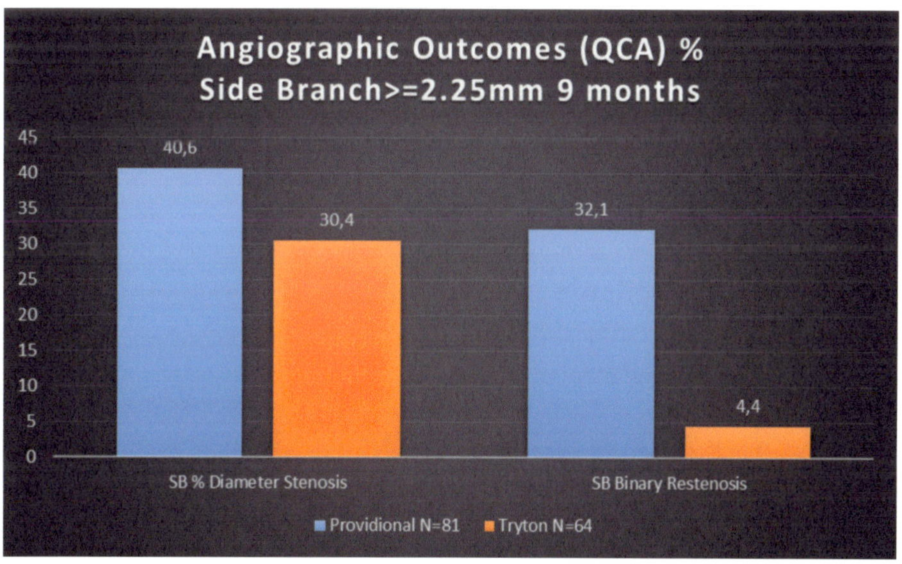

Figure 5. QCA outcomes in TRYTON subanalysis (Genereux et al. Catheter Cardiovasc Interv. 2015).

Confirmatory study		Randomized trial > = 2.25mm	
Endpoints %	**TRYTON** **N = 133**	**TRYTON** **N = 146**	**Provisional** **N = 143**
Death			
Procedural	0% (0.0)	0% (0.0)	0% (0.0)
30-day	0% (0.0)	0% (0.0)	0% (0.0)
Myocardial infarction			
Procedural (3xCKMB)	10.5% (14/133)	9.2% (13/141)	12.1% (17/141)
Procedural (5× CKMB)	4.5% (7/133)	3.4% (4/118)	6.8% (7/103)
30-day	10.8% (14/130)	8.2% (12/146)	11.9% (17/143)
Stent thrombosis	0% (0.0)	0.7% ()1/146	0.0% (0/143)

Table 1. Procedural and 30-day follow-up.

had an SB ≥2.25 mm. The primary endpoint of TVF was numerically lower in the Tryton group compared with the provisional group (11.3% vs. 15.6%, P = 0.38). No difference among the rates of clinically driven target vessel revascularization or cardiac death was seen. In-segment percent diameter stenosis of the SB was significantly lower (10.2%) in the Tryton group compared with the provisional group. In conclusion, TRYTON trial cohort of SB ≥2.25 mm supports the safety and efficacy of the Tryton SB stent compared with a provisional stenting strategy in the treatment of bifurcation lesions involving large SBs [4] (**Figures 4** and **5**).

TRYTON confirmatory study rationale was to prospectively confirm the safety (periprocedural MI) of the Tryton dedicated bifurcation stent in the treatment of true bifurcation lesions involving large side branches (>2.25 mm by QCA analysis). The angiographic inclusion criteria were the same. The study included 28 investigational centers with 12-month enrolment. Procedural and 30-day follow-up are given in **Table 1**.

4. AXXESS stent

Another bifurcation stent is AXXESS.

Axxess is self-expanding nickel-titanium alloy; it has conical shape and proximal and distal gold markers, facilitating implantation. The device is Biolimus A9 coated using a bioabsorbable polymer matrix in a dose of 22 mg/mm of stent length. The strut thickness is 0.15 mm and the drug release rate is 70% in 30 days, remaining 30% released in <6 months with polymer absorption 6–9 months.

There are three models of the stent—11 and 14 mm in length with reference diameter 2.75–3.25 mm. The maximal proximal and distal stent diameters are 3.75 and 6 mm, respectively. For reference diameter 3.25–3.75, the maximal proximal and distal stent diameters are 4.25 and 6.5 mm. The delivery system is covered sheath, that is, rapid-exchange delivery catheter. It is 5 Fr of higher compatible.

http://dx.doi.org/10.5772/intechopen.82573

The goal of stent placement is to cover the proximal lesion segment as well as the ostium of the side branch and distal patent vessel without compromising access to the side branch. It is accomplished if two markers - in 1 branch and 1 is in the other. Axxess provides convenient placement marker for additional distal stents (**Figure 6**).

Stent implantation—the AXXESS stent is advanced so it is astride the carina and is pushed further forward as far as it will go. Implantation steps: a wire is placed in each branch; the stent is advanced to the most angulated branch, and the distal stent markers are aligned with the carina; the self-expanding distal struts partially expand as the sheath is partially withdrawn after which the partially expanded stent in the main branch is advanced to cover the bifurcation (**Figure 7**).

4.1. Clinical studies

There is a growing body of literature that supports the use of the AXXESS system in the treatment of coronary bifurcation lesions. The first-in-man AXXESS Plus trial reported results at 6 months in 139 patients who underwent implantation across 13 centers, with low rates of TLR (7.5%) and late-lumen loss (0.09 mm). There was a low rate of periprocedural complications (MACE rate 5% (n = 7), non-Q wave MI 4.3% (n = 6)), with a late-stent thrombosis rate of 2.1% (three patients, two of whom associated with premature cessation of antiplatelet therapy) [6].

The following DIVERGE Trial was a prospective, single-arm, multicenter trial. Any type of bifurcation lesion was included with significant SB larger than 2.25 mm and PV-SB angulation <70° (**Figure 8**).

About 302 patients in 16 clinical sites in Europe, Australia, and New Zealand were included. Clinical follow-up at the first, sixth, ninth month, and after that yearly up to fifth year was completed.

First endpoint was MACE at 9 months, with secondary end points and 12 months and 2-, 3-, 4- and 5-year death, cardiac death, MI-Q and non-Q, TLR, TVR, stent thrombosis at 30 days, 6,

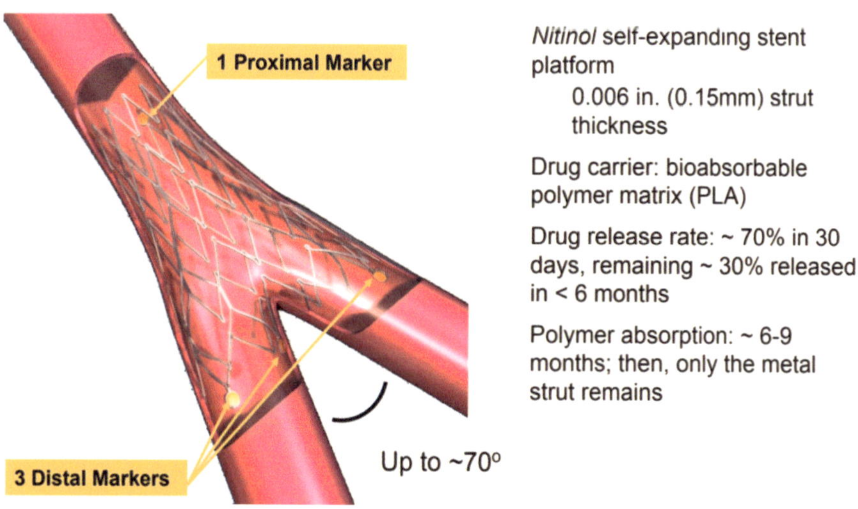

Figure 6. Axxess structure. Source: Rizik et al. [5].

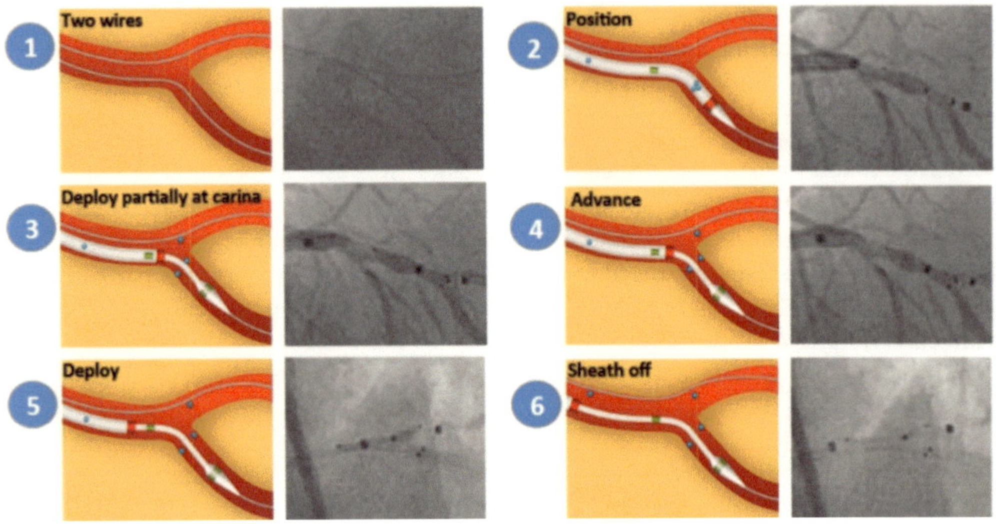

Figure 7. Axxess deployment sequence.

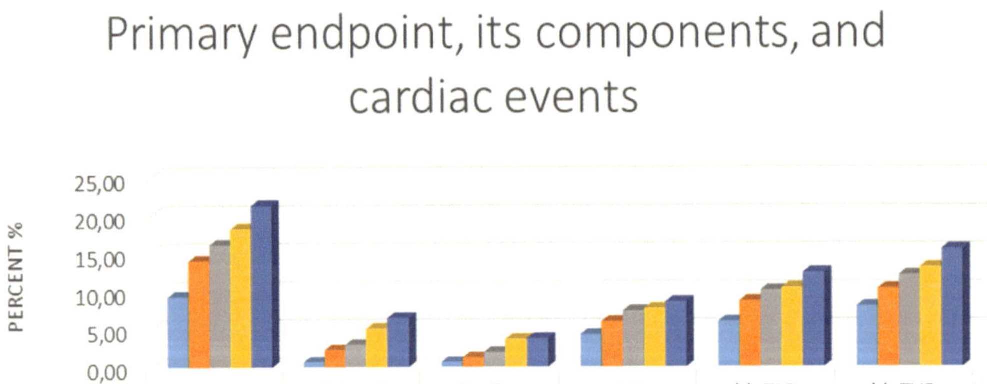

	MACE	All Death	Cardiac Death	MI	id- TLR	id- TVR
12 Months	9,30	0,70	0,70	4,30	6,00	8,00
2 Years	14,00	2,30	1,30	6,00	8,70	10,30
3 Years	16,10	3,00	2,00	7,40	10,10	12,10
4 Years	18,20	5,10	3,70	7,70	10,40	13,10
5 Years	21,30	6,50	3,80	8,60	12,40	15,50

Figure 8. DIVERGE trial: 5-year outcomes.

9, and 12 months and 2, 3, 4, and 5 years. The angiographic secondary end points were in-stent restenosis and late loss at 9 months. DAPT for 12 months was recommended. About 77.4% of all patients were with true bifurcations with predominating Medina 1:1:1.

Axxess only was used in 12.3%; Axxess with PV stenting in 17.7%, Axxess with SB stenting in 4%, and stenting of the two branches was present in 64.7%. In general, side branch stent was used in 68.7%.

http://dx.doi.org/10.5772/intechopen.82573

9 – month QCA results			
At follow-up		**Parent vessel N = 140**	**Side branch N = 140**
Late loss (mm)	In-stent LL (Axxess only)	0.18 ± 0.49	-
	In-stent LL (all stents)	0.29 ± 0.50	0.29 ± 0.45
	In-lesion LL	0.20 ± 0.41	0.17 ± 0.34
Restenosis per vessel	In-stent LL (Axxess only)	0.7%	-
	In-stent (Cypher)	2.3%	4.8%
	In-lesion restenosis (all stents + edges)	3.6%	4.3%
Overall bifurcation restenosis	In-stent PV+SB	5% (7/140)	
	In-stent or edges PV+SB	6.4% (9/140)	

Table 2. QCA results.

Nine-month QCA results are presented in **Table 2** [7, 8].

Another study evaluating Axxess in bifurcation treatment is COBRA [8]. It compares Axxess + DES versus culotte with EES. OCT stent and lumen area at ninth month are compared. The percentage of uncovered struts in each bifurcation segment at 9 months (primary end-point) was similar between groups. Five-year clinical follow-up was available for all patients and included major adverse cardiac events [MACE; a composite of cardiac death, myocardial infarction (MI) and ischemia-driven target lesion revascularization (TLR)], target-vessel (TVR) and non-target-vessel revascularization (non-TVR), non-TLR, and stent thrombosis. At

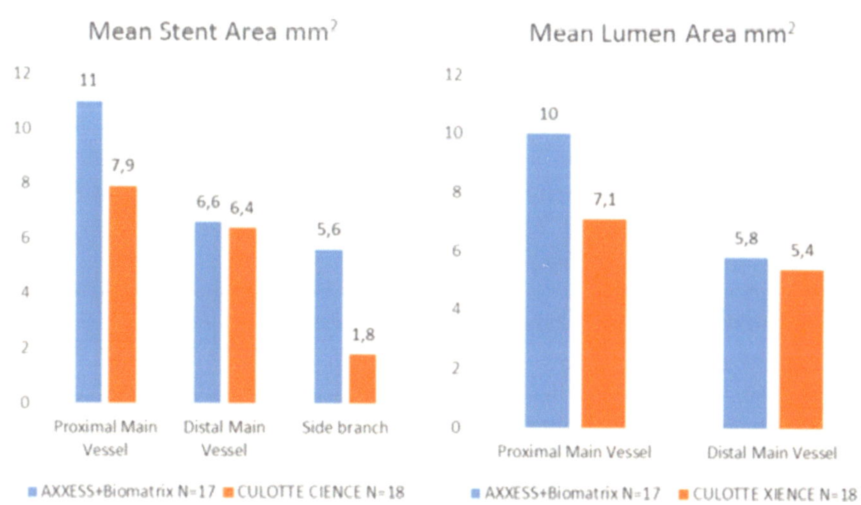

Figure 9. COBRA trial results at 9 months.

5 years, in the culotte group, one patient had undergone TLR and another suffered a clinical MI, resulting in 10% MACE versus none in the Axxess group. TVR (5 vs. 10%, P = 0.54) and non-TVR (5 vs. 20%, P = 0.39) rates were similar between the Axxess and culotte groups, respectively. There was no stent thrombosis (**Figure 9**).

In conclusion, Axxess is a self-expanding coated device with positive results in bifurcation lesions, including complex morphology. It has relatively high profile, and frequently multiple stents are used in cases of double stenting. There is some proof or larger luminal gain in the carina segment. Prospective data support its use in complex coronary bifurcations; however, its use has yet to be studied in a large-scale randomized controlled trial.

5. BiOSS stent

The BiOSS stent (Balton, Warsaw, Poland)—Bifurcation Optimisation Stent System was created and firstly used in 2008. It has three generations. At first, it started as bare metal BiOSS stent, then drug-eluting stents—BiOSS Expert in 2010; then in 2012, BiOSS LIM was introduced. Recently, in 2018, the last generation BiOSS LIM C was tested in man.

5.1. The stent design

All generations of BiOSS stent have the same primary design. As it is delivered by one 0.014 guidewire through rapid-exchange system with five French guiding catheter, it makes BIOSS no different than the other conventional stents. The difference comes with the strut and balloon design.

We know from the Murray's law (see **Figure 10**) of bifurcations that there is difference between main vessel and side branch diameters. In plain words, the bigger the side branch, the bigger the difference of proximal and distal part of the main vessel. When we plan to stent a bifurcation, we should choose a stent that has the diameter of the distal part of the main vessel, and after implantation, we do a proximal optimization—to dilate a bigger balloon at the proximal part (above carina) to keep the stent conformation as the natural anatomic structure.

In case we choose stent size 1:1 in diameter to the proximal part of the main vessel it will overstretch the distal part thus moving the carina and plaque to the orifice of the side branch and compromising the blood flow. Secondly, the conventional stents, even with open cell design, will have struts at the side branch orifice.

Main difference between those different generation of stents are the material (BiOSS Expert and LIM being the same design stainless steel 140-μm struts and BiOSS LIM C made from cobalt-chromium alloy 70-μm struts) and different drug (first-generation BiOSS Expert eluted paclitaxel and the next BiOSS LIM and LIM C eluted sirolimus). So there is huge difference between them as 140 μm may provoke arterial wall injury and lead neointimal proliferation and thinner struts may facilitate endothelialization [8]. The other important difference is the

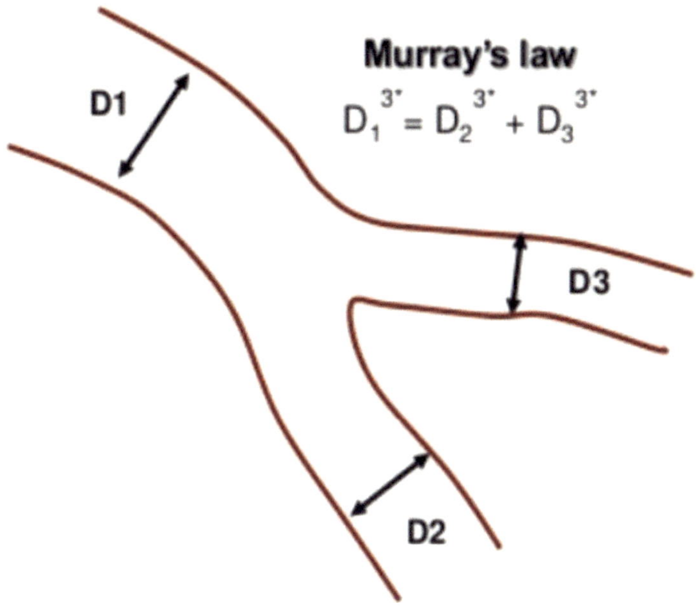

Figure 10. Visualization of Murray's law.

drug that is eluted paclitaxel in BiOSS Expert and sirolimus in LIM and LIM C as it was shown that sirolimus decreased the rates of MACE and TLR [9, 10].

5.2. How the stent design of BiOSS comes to tackle these problems?

The stent is made of two parts—proximal and distal with two small connecting struts at the middle zone (0.9–1.5 mm in length). The proximal part of the stent has a larger diameter than the distal one—the ratio is 1.15–1.3. Proximal diameters vary from 3.25 to 4.5 mm and the distal ones from 2.5 to 3.75; the stent length is 15, 18, and 23 mm. The proximal part is always a bit shorter than the distal one (average 1 mm). So, for instance, the smallest stent is 2.5 × 3.25 mm in diameter—distal and proximal part and the largest one is 3.75 × 4.5 mm, and there are four varieties between them with 0.5–0.75 difference in proximal and distal diameters (2.75 × 3.5 mm; 3.0 × 3.5 mm; 3 × 3.75 mm; 3.5 × 4.25 mm). So with three different lengths, it makes a total of 18 combinations. The stent is delivered on a bottle-shaped balloon (Bottle, Balton, Poland), allowing bigger proximal and smaller distal diameter when inflated. It is semicomplaint balloon with nominal pressure of 10 atm and burst pressure of 18 atm (**Figures 11** and **12**).

The stent has three markers: two at both ends and one in the middle. The markers at both ends are like every other stent—they show proximal and distal ends of the device. The midmarker shows the proximal end of the distal (smaller) part of the stent—it should be positioned exactly at the carina as shown in **Figure 13**. So this placement helps to keep the natural anatomic proportions (bigger proximal part, smaller distal) and keep same carina confirmation—it has no carina displacement because the lateral force from proximal stretching counterbalances with the medial force from distal stretching. The other important design virtue is that there are no struts at the opening of the side branch.

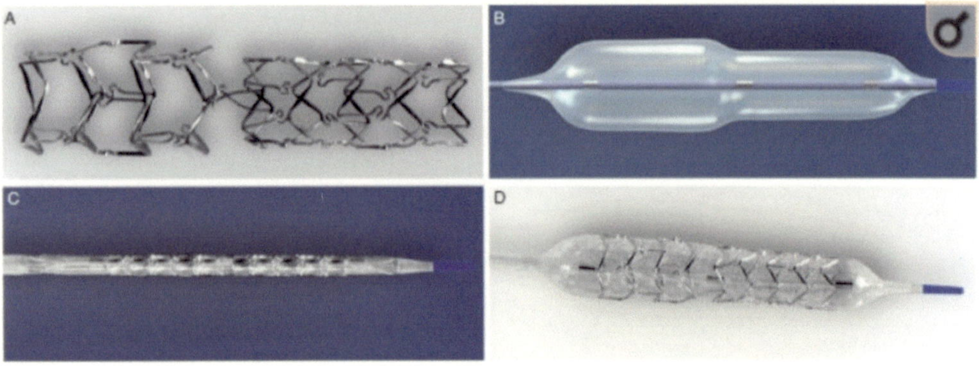

Figure 11. (A) Expanded stent; (B) stent balloon only; (C) stent system not expended; (D) expanded stent system. Source: Gil et al. [11].

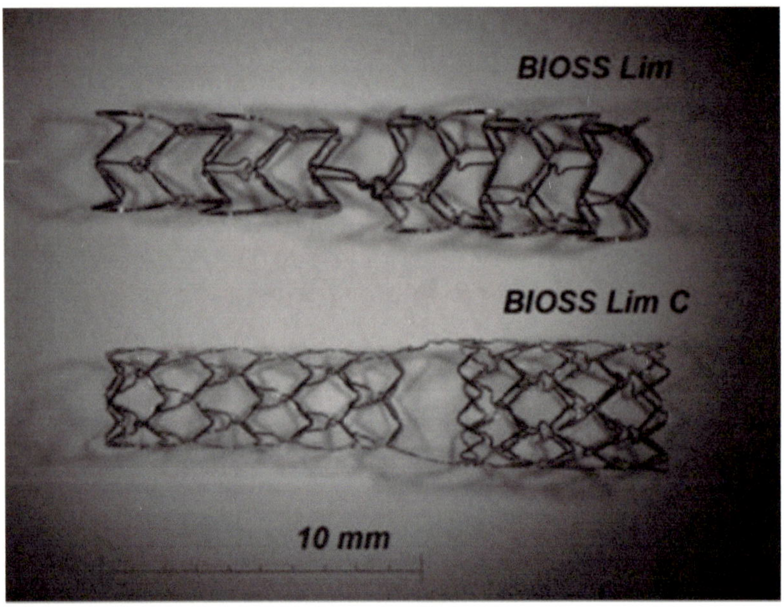

Figure 12. BIOSS Lim and BIOSS Lim C stents. Source: Gil et al. [12].

An IVUS study showed that BiOSS stent provides better access to the SB in comparison with the conventional drug-eluting stents. There was significantly bigger orifice length found in the BiOSS group—a parameter, which represents the access to the SB [13]. The analysis of the plaque, lumen, and vessel areas shows that BiOSS stent design spares the proximal optimization technique (POT), which is strongly recommended by the European Bifurcation Club [14]. But this imposes the question whether no struts at the carina could predispose to restenosis. This issue was addressed in the IVUS study and showed that the carina actually had the least neointimal burden during follow-up [15]. This study also showed that sirolimus was better than paclitaxel in rates of neointimal hyperplasia.

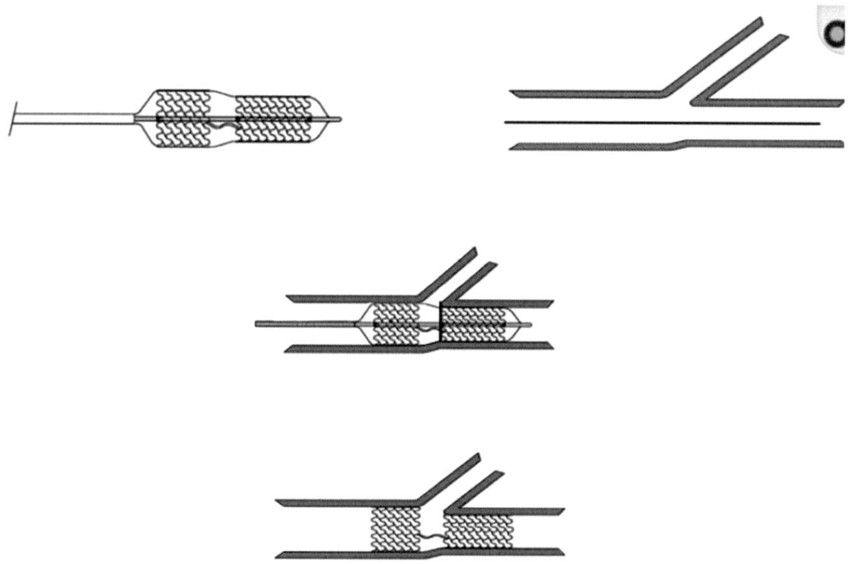

Figure 13. Visualization of stent positioning. Source: Gil et al. [12].

5.3. What are the results when comparing BiOSS stent versus conventional DES in treating bifurcation lesions?

Two randomized multicenter trials compared BiOSS Expert and LIM versus conventional drug-eluting stents—POLBOS I (2010–2013) and POLBOS II (2012–2013).

They have published results at 12 and 48 months of follow-up.

POLBOS I (n = 243) study compared BiOSS Expert (paclitaxel) stent versus conventional DES—paclitaxel, sirolimus, everolimus, zotarolimus, and tacrolimus stents (LucChopin2, Xience, Promus, Cypher, Prolim, Orsiro, Biomime, Biomatrix, Resolute Integrity, and Optima). POT balloons were advised but left to operator discretion. Kissing was left to operator discretion in BiOSS group, and in DES group, there was second randomization for kissing balloons.

At 12 months of follow up, the cumulative incidence of MACE was similar in both groups 13.3% in BiOSS vs. 12.2% in DES. There were also no significant differences in cardiac-related death (0 in BiOSS vs. 1.6% in DES), myocardial infarctions (1.6% in BiOSS vs. 3.2% in DES), and stent thrombosis (0.8% in BiOSS vs. 0 in DES). Target vessel revascularizations were significantly higher in BiOSS group 15.8% vs. 9.7% in DES group. Target lesion revascularizations were also significantly higher in BiOSS group 11.5% vs. 7.3% in DES group.

POLBOS II (n = 202) compared the next-generation BiOSS LIM (sirolimus) stent vs. regular DES (same as above). POT and kissing were left to operator discretion in BiOSS group and POT to operator discretion but kissing randomized in DES group. At 12 months, there were no significant differences in MACE (11.8% in BiOSS vs. 15% in DES), death (1% in BiOSS vs. 3% DES), MI (1.9 vs. 3%), TLR (9.8% in BiOSS vs. 9% in DES), and TVR (13.7% in BiOSS vs.

12% in DES). Final kissing was associated with significantly less TLR only in BiOSS group (5.9 vs. 11.8%, $p < 0.05$), but POT technique was associated with less TLR in both groups (in BiOSS 5.3% vs. 12.5% $p < 0.05$ and in DES group 2.9% vs. 25% $p < 0.01$).

When analyzed POLBOS I and II at 48 months, there were no statistical differences in terms of MACE (DES vs. BiOSS: 18.8 vs. 19.8%, $p = 0.64$), TLR (12.1 vs. 15.3%, $p = 0.34$), MI (4.5 vs. 2.1%, $p = 0.72$), or cardiac death (2.2 vs. 1.8%, $p = 0.81$) between DES and BiOSS groups.

5.4. Why one should use BiOSS stent if the long-term results are the same?

Implanting BiOSS stent will not spare you the proximal optimization or the kissing balloons if there is a need for such techniques. In theory, it will leave the SB ostium open, thus making it easier to reach with a wire and go through it with a balloon for a kissing. In case you need two-stent technique, there will be less struts at the carina and easier to go through with a second stent.

So in our opinion, BiOSS stent makes treating of bifurcation lesion simpler and sometimes cheaper (sparing a smaller balloon for opening the struts to the side branch in order to reach with a bigger one for kissing).

5.5. What are the pitfalls in implanting BiOSS stent?

In our opinion, there are two main issues when implanting BiOSS stent. The first is when you have long lesion that incudes bifurcation. Consider that longest BiOSS is 23 mm in length with approximately 46/50% length in proximal and distal length, so having a longer than 12 mm proximal or distal lesions means that if you are planning to use BiOSS, you will need at least two stents, one regular DES and one BiOSS; in this case, implanting just one long regular DES and doing proximal optimization is more suitable.

The second is that when implanting BiOSS stent, it is of crucial matter to find very good projections where carina is seen, because you have to place the middle marker at the ostium of the main branch (**Figure 14**).

Figure 14. Correctly positioned stent (angio).

Implanting the stent beyond the carina will compromise the side branch ostium; in the other case, implanting the stent too much proximal to the carina will not have these adverse effects in the side branch but will leave struts at the carina.

In conclusion, BiOSS stent should be considered a good choice for treating bifurcation lesions, intended for one- or two-stent strategy.

6. Nile concept

Minvasys offers one of the current stent solutions for bifurcation stenting. First approved stent from Nile family is Nile CroCo, which takes CE brand in 2005. Nile CroCo presents the basic Minvasys concept of bifurcation stenting. Future generations of dedicated stents are based on Nile CroCo.

6.1. Nile CroCo

Nile CroCo stent is based on cobalt-chromium bare metal platform. The stent consists of three segments. Proximal segment includes 7–9 cells (depending on stent size), the medial segment includes 8–10 cells, and the distal segment includes 6–8 cells (**Figure 15**). This distribution ensures same metal to artery ratio (between 10.3 and 14.6%) [16] along entire bifurcation, which is important for optimal stent apposition. Stent thickness of Nile CroCo platform is 73 μm. Two stent length are offered—18 and 24 mm; three diameters for main branch balloon (2.5, 3.0, and 3.5 mm) and three diameters for side branch balloon (2.0, 2.5, and 3.0 mm) are offered. There are seven stents with different MB and SB diameters (as follows: 2.5–2.0, 3.0–2.0, 3.0–2.5, 3.5–2.5, 3.5–3.0, 2.5–2.5, and 3.0–3.0 mm), each of them proposed in two lengths (18 and 24 mm).

Stent delivery system integrates two monorail balloons: one for the side branch and one for the main branch. It requires 6.0F guiding catheter for stent delivery, and two 0.014-inch guidewires, previously positioned in MB and SB. Both balloons have similar characteristics with nominal pressure 8 atm and rated burst pressure 14 atm (**Figure 16**).

Cobalt-chromium stent platform is mounted on main branch balloon. The system also contains side branch catheter tip. Side branch balloon is located proximally from the stent. Both balloon catheters are rapid exchange. In order to prevent entanglement of two balloon shafts, during system delivery, there is autorelease sheath. The system is equipped with five roentgen-positive markers—three of them located on MB balloon—proximal, distal, and medial. Medial marker is located exactly on the bifurcation. There are two additional markers, pointing proximal and distal parts of SB balloon.

Despite the fact that every dedicated bifurcation stent proposes a unique approach to bifurcation lesion, Nile system allows provisional T-stenting in the A category, according to MADS classification. Provisional stenting strategy is recommended as the first-line approach by many modern consensuses.

Stenting procedure (**Figure 17**). The stenting procedure begins with placement of two guidewires distally in the main branch and side branch (step 1). Predilatation of MB and SB (if stenosis seems to be significant) is crucial for seamlessly stent delivery. Optimal stent size must be selected according to distal diameters of MB and SB. The system must be introduced on the both rapid-exchange balloon catheters. After that, the system is pushed through the guiding catheter. During the advancement, autorelease sheath must be released. Two monorail balloon catheters are advanced until distal part of the stent crosses through stenosis in the main branch. When the midsegment of the stent is positioned on the carina, and the tip of SB balloon catheter is in the proximal part of the SB (step 2), the system will stop and the operator will feel resistance. At this moment, the middle roentgen positive marker must be exactly at the level of carina (shown with a narrow at step 2). In this way, the operator is maximally facilitated in optimal positioning the stent because it can use guidewires as well as the radiopaque marker and tactile sensation.

In about 40% of cases, twisting of guidewires may occur. This can be easily solved by retrieving the system in the guiding catheter and repositioning one of the guidewires.

After optimal stent positioning, the MB balloon is inflated, providing stent implantation in the main branch (step 3). After this step, the medium "strutless" part of the stent is positioned exactly at the level of bifurcation. Next step is advancement of the SB balloon catheter into SB ostium (step 4). This can be achieved easily, because of two facts. First of all, the SB guidewire is not jailed, so there is no need to recross wires. Furthermore, there is a "defect" in the struts, at the level of carina that allows balloon advancement. The next step (step 5) is kissing, using both balloons, integrated in the system. Because of the special SB balloon shape, overextension of the proximal segment of the bifurcation is avoided. After the removal of delivery system (step 6), both guidewires stay positioned into main branch and side branch. This made implantation of additional stent (only if necessary) very easy.

This concept of stent implantation is preserved in next two generations of Nile stents—Nile PAX and Nile SIR.

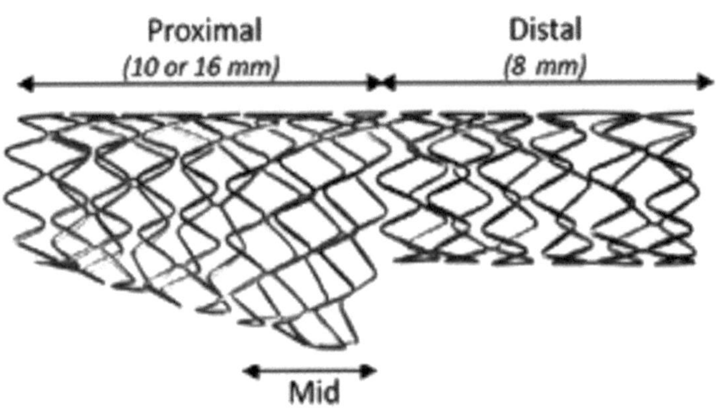

Figure 15. Nile CroCo structure. Source: [17].

http://dx.doi.org/10.5772/intechopen.82573

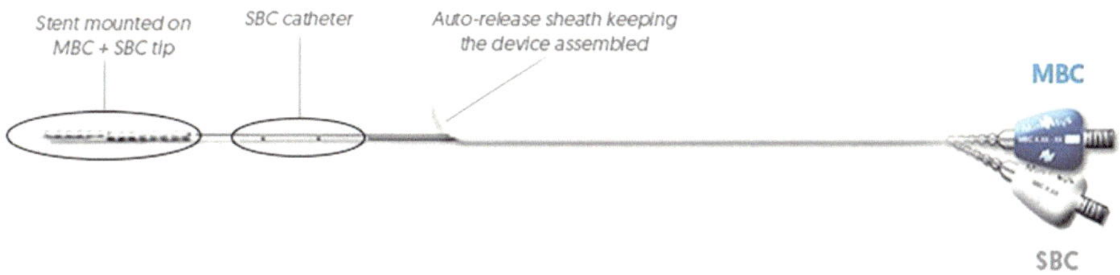

Figure 16. Scheme of delivery system. Source: [17].

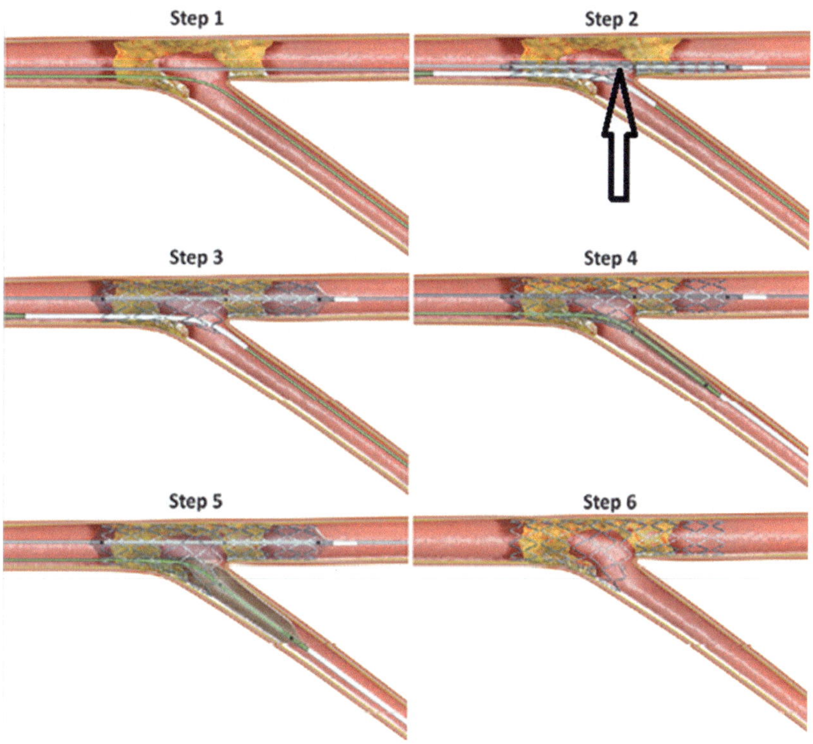

Figure 17. Stenting procedure step-by-step. Source: [17].

Bruno Garcia Del Blanco et al. reported the results of a series of 151 patients treated successfully by implantation of Nile CroCo stent [18]. Success in stent positioning and implantation was reported in 99% of patients. Radial approach was used in 75% of patients. In more than 80% of patients, 6F introducer and guiding catheter was enough. Significant lesion at the ostium of the SB was reported in 73% of patients. A kissing inflation with the system was performed in almost all (95%). In 19% of cases, additional stent was implanted in MB, while in 10% of cases, additional stent was implanted in SB. Among 138 patients with a complete follow-up at 6 months, the MACE rate was 14% and the TLR was 7.2%, despite the fact that the patient profile being relatively severe, including 55 patients with myocardial infarction <24 h. Guidewire twisting—as mentioned earlier—requiring repositioning was noted in 33% of cases.

6.2. Nile PAX

In 2009, next-generation (**Figure 18**) bifurcation stent gets CE brand approval. Stent structure, stent sizes, and delivery system are the same as in Nile CroCo. The stent was made by same cobalt-chromium alloy with similar metal to artery ratio (between 10 and 15%). Strut thickness is 73 µm, but in Nile PAX, there are additional 5-µm polymer-free coatings with paclitaxel only on the abluminal surface in crystallized form. Drug concentration is 2.5 µg/mm^2, and based on manufacturer's data, whole drug is released 45 days after stent implantation.

Stent delivery system and the steps of stent implantation are actually the same as described for Nile CroCo stents. Because of that, we will repeat the steps, using our real clinical case for visualization.

We present 68-year-old female with stable angina pectoris and bifurcation LM stenosis (Medina 0:1:1) (**Figure 19**).

We placed two 0.014 inch guidewires in MB and SB and made predilatation of MB with NC balloon 2.0/20 mm (please note that LCx is chosen for MB). Stent positioning with central marker at the level of carina is shown in **Figure 20**.

The balloon for the SB postdilatation may be seen in guiding catheter on this step. After angiographic verification of optimal stent apposition, MB balloon was inflated (**Figure 21**). Final kissing was made, using both balloons incorporated in system, and the final result is visualized in **Figure 22**.

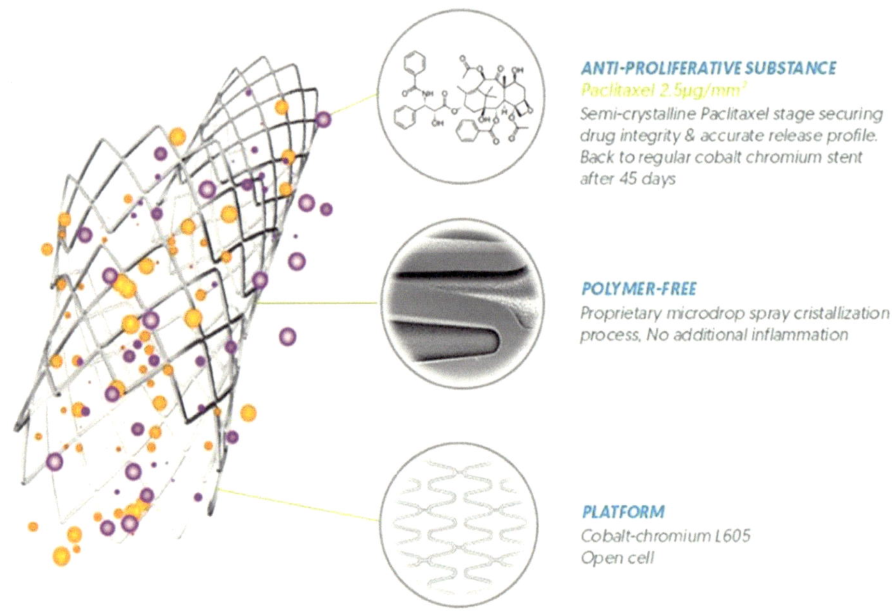

Figure 18. Nile PAX stent. Source: Owned by Acibadem City Clinic.

http://dx.doi.org/10.5772/intechopen.82573

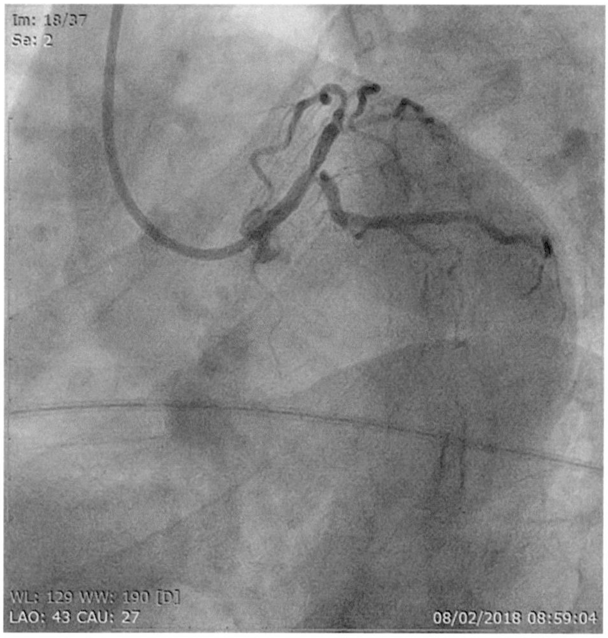

Figure 19. Stenosis before the beginning of the procedure. Source: Owned by Acibadem City Clinic.

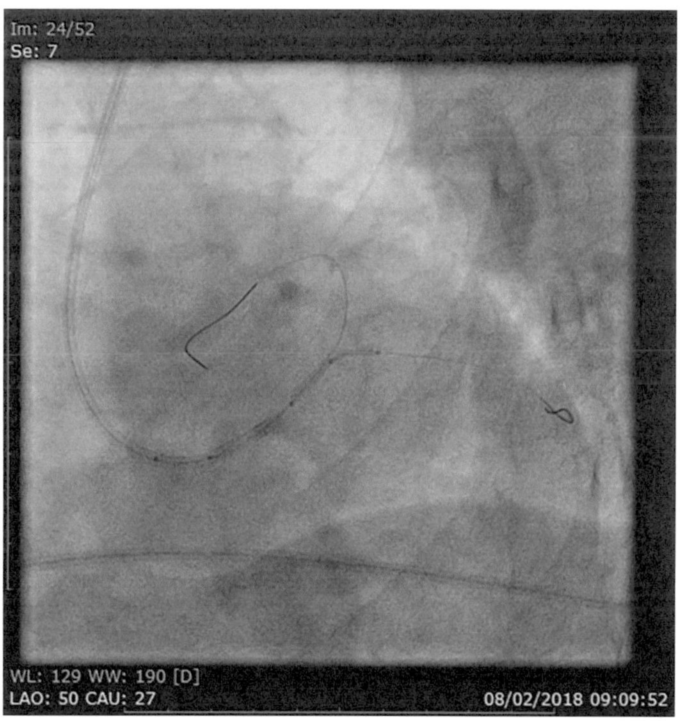

Figure 20. Stent positioning. Source: Owned by Acibadem City Clinic.

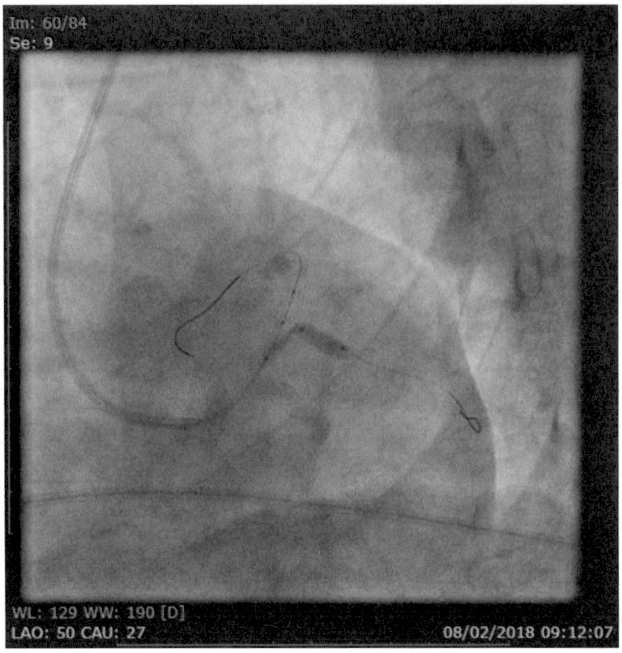

Figure 21. Inflation of MB balloon. Source: Owned by Acibadem City Clinic.

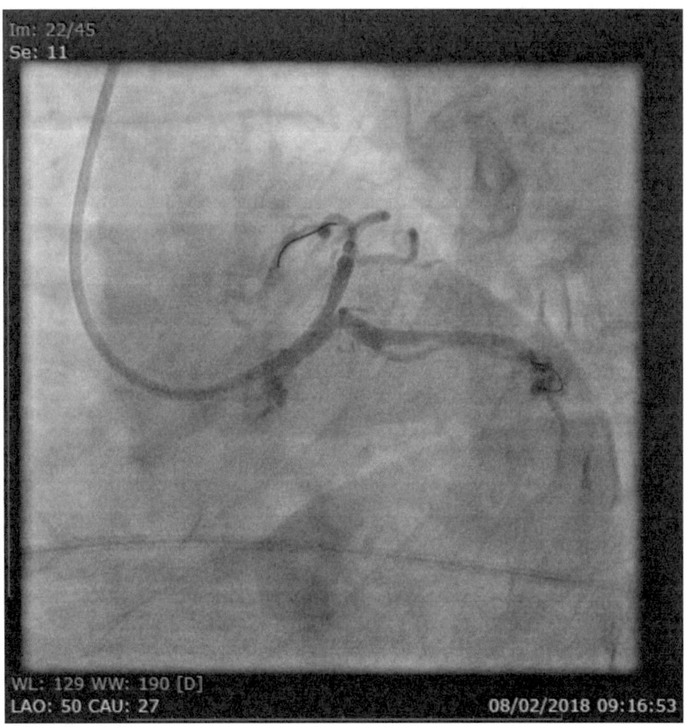

Figure 22. Final result. Source: [20].

http://dx.doi.org/10.5772/intechopen.82573

In 2012, results from a big trial with Nile PAX stent were published [19]. The trial is multicenter, including 101 patients from Europe and Brazil. Our team is part of this study. Procedural success and 30-day follow-up data of the paclitaxel-eluting version (Nile PAX) were presented. In 80% of cases, the LAD-diagonal branch bifurcation was the target lesion with 62% also having an SB lesion. In total, 102 lesions were treated, of which 62% had a stenosis on each of the main or side branches. Procedural success was achieved in 97% of cases. An additional stent was implanted in the SB in 25% of cases. Longer-term (9-month) clinical follow-up data of this study were presented at EuroPCR 2011 (by Bruno Garcia). The rate of restenosis was 13.9% in the MB, 12.8% in the SB, and a total of 18.6% in the bifurcation, which led to a TLR of 12.6% with only one myocardial infarction reported.

In order to reduce the rate of SB restenosis (12.8%) found in the Nile PAX trial, a new Nile PAX study with systematic use of a paclitaxel-eluting balloon (Danubio; Minvasys) in the SB at the end of the procedure shows only 2% rate of restenosis.

6.3. Nile SIR

Last generation of Minvasys Nile family is Nile SIR dedicated bifurcation stent. It is based on the same conception as Nile CroCo and Nile PAX but covered by sirolimus as antiproliferative drug. Sirolimus is deposited with biodegradable polymer on abluminal stent surface with concentration 1.4 $\mu g/mm^2$. About 85% of the drug is expected to be eluted within 48 days after implantation, and complete reversion to BMS is expected within 180 days.

The active drug is deposed on abluminal stent surface on two layers (**Figure 23**). First layer (A) contains sirolimus, poly-L lactic acid, poly(lactic-co-glycolic) acid, and polyvinylpyrrolidone. It is located between stent strut and layer B. Layer B is water soluble, contains polyvinylpyrrolidone, and had only protective function.

Between 2013 and 2014 in India, 37 patients with symptomatic bifurcation stenosis were treated by implantation of Nile SIR and followed up. Most of the patients had LAD-DIAGONAL stenosis (74%), and 26% had LCx-OM stenosis. Stable angina at admission was reported in 64.9%, and the rest was with unstable angina pectoris. There were no procedural complications or adverse cardiac events till discharge. In 27% of patients, there was additional stent implanted at the MB level,

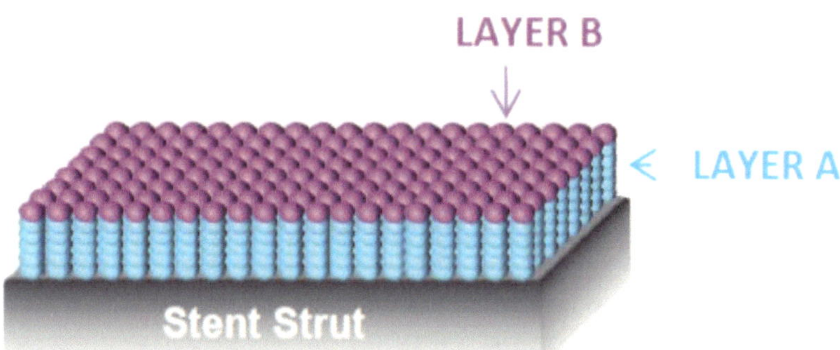

Figure 23. Drug deposal on the stent.

and 3% of patients had additional stent implanted in SB. During 6-month clinical follow-up, there was no MACE reported. Three of the patients were died from noncardiac reason. Angiographic follow-up was done in 15 of these patients. In-stent late-lumen loss was reported as follows: on the proximal MB level 0.15 ± 0.15, on the distal MB level 0.16 ± 0.29, and on the SB level 0.26 ± 0.41.

In our center, 42 patients with bifurcation LM stenosis were treated in the past 2 years. About 52.94% of patients had stable angina and 47.06% with acute MI (including one patient with STEMI). Based on the Medina classification, bifurcation lesions were type 1:1:1 in 33.82%, type 1:0:1 in 20.59%, and type 0:1:1 in 11.76% patients. Procedural success was achieved in all patients. According to center protocol, clinical follow-up was done on the first month. Control angiography with intravascular ultrasound was done on the sixth month. Twenty-four (57.14%) patients were followed up angiographically. We observed two MACE (4.76%)—one patient died before FU and one in-stent restenosis at the SB level. The measures of the late-lumen loss were 0.22 ± 0.38, 0.29 ± 0.34, and 0.18 ± 0.31 mm for the main branch proximal, distal, and side branch, respectively.

Conflict of interest

There is no conflict of interest to declare.

Author details

Ivo Petrov, Iveta Tasheva*, Jivka Stoykova, Liubomir Dosev, Zoran Stankov and Petar Polomski

*Address all correspondence to: iveta_t@yahoo.com

Acibadem City Clinic Cardiovascular Center, Sofia, Bulgaria

References

[1] Arora RR et al. Catheterization and Cardiovascular Diagnosis. 1989;**18**:210-212

[2] Généreux P, Kumsars I, Lesiak M. A randomized trial of a dedicated bifurcation stent versus provisional stenting in the treatment of coronary bifurcation lesions. Journal of the American College of Cardiology

[3] Genereux P. TRYTON Pivotal: Randomized Trial and Confirmatory Study

[4] Généreux P, Kini A, Lesiak M. Outcomes of a dedicated stent in coronary bifurcations with large side branches: A subanalysis of the randomized TRYTON bifurcation study. Catheterization and Cardiovascular Interventions. 2016;**87**(7):1231-1241. DOI: 10.1002/ccd.26240

[5] Rizik DG, Klassen KJ, Hermiller JB. Bifurcation coronary artery disease: Current techniques and future directions (Part 2). The Journal of invasive cardiology. 2008;**20**(3):135-141

[6] Rawlins J, Din J, Talwar S, O'Kane P. AXXESS™ stent: Delivery indications and outcomes. Interventional Cardiology. 2015;**10**(2):85-89. DOI: 10.15420/icr.2015.10.2.85

[7] Verheye S, Agostoni P, Dubois CL, et al. 9-month clinical, angiographic, and intravascular ultrasound results of a prospective evaluation of the Axxess self-expanding biolimus A9-eluting stent in coronary bifurcation lesions: The DIVERGE (drug-eluting stent intervention for treating side branches effectively) study. Journal of the American College of Cardiology. 2009;**53**(12):1031-1039. DOI: 10.1016/j.jacc.2008.12.012

[8] Pache J, Kastrati A, Mehilli J, et al. Intracoronary stenting and angiographic results: Strut thickness effect on restenosis outcome (ISAR-STEREO-2) trial. Journal of the American College of Cardiology. 2003;**41**(8):1283-1288

[9] Kong J, Liu P, Fan X, et al. Long-term outcomes of paclitaxel-eluting versus sirolimus-eluting stent for percutaneous coronary intervention: A meta-analysis. Journal of the College of Physicians and Surgeons–Pakistan. 2017;**27**(7):432-439. DOI: 2659

[10] Minvasys Website. Available from: http://www.minvasys.com/fr/ bifurcation-stents/nile-croco.php [Accessed: December 14, 2018]

[11] Gil RG, Bil J, Vassilev D. The BiOSS stent. EuroIntervention. 2015;**11**:V153-V154

[12] Gil RJ, Bil J, Kern A, Pawłowski T. First-in-man study of dedicated bifurcation cobalt-chromium sirolimus-eluting stent BiOSS LIM C®—Three-month results. Kardiologia Polska. 2018;**76**(2):464-470. DOI: 10.5603/KP.a2017.0226

[13] Gil RJ, Michalek A, Bil J. Comparative analysis of lumen enlargement mechanisms achieved with bifurcation dedicated stent BiOSS® and classical coronary stent implantations by means of provisional side branch stenting strategy—The intravascular ultrasound study. The International Journal of Cardiovascular Imaging. 2013;**29**(8):1667-1676. DOI: 10.1007/s10554-013-0264-0

[14] Lassen JF, Holm NR, Banning A, Burzotta F, Lefèvre T, Chieffo A, et al. Percutaneous coronary intervention for coronary bifurcation disease: 11th consensus document from the European Bifurcation Club. EuroIntervention. 2016;**12**(1):38-46. DOI: 10.4244/EIJV12I1A7

[15] Gil RJ, Bil J, Costa RA, Gil KE, Vassiliev D. 12-month intravascular ultrasound observations from BiOSS® first-in-man studies. The International Journal of Cardiovascular Imaging. 2016;**32**(9):1339-1347. DOI: 10.1007/s10554-016-0926-9

[16] Ughi GJ, Verjans J, Fard AM. Dual modality intravascular optical coherence tomography (OCT) and near-infrared fluorescence (NIRF) imaging: A fully automated algorithm for the distance-calibration of NIRF signal intensity for quantitative molecular imaging. The International Journal of Cardiovascular Imaging. 2015;**31**(2):259-268

[17] http://www.minvasys.com/fr/bifurcation-stents/nile-pax.php

[18] Garcia del Blanco G, Bellera Gotarda N, Martí G, et al. Clinical and procedural evaluation of the Nile Croco dedicated stent for bifurcation. Results of one center initial experience with the first 151 consecutive non-selected patients. EuroIntervention. Abstract Book; 2011. p. H45

[19] Costa RA, Abizaid A, Abizaid AS, Garcia del Blanco B, et al. BIPAX investigators. Procedural and early clinical outcomes of patients with de novo coronary bifurcation lesions treated with the novel Nile PAX dedicated bifurcation polymer-free paclitaxel coated stents: Results from the prospective, multicentre, non-randomised BIPAX clinical trial. EuroIntervention. 2012;7:1301-1309

[20] https://www.minvasys.com/nile-sir-technology.php

Section 3

Angiography for Peripheral Arterial Diseases

Chapter 6

Angiography for Renal Artery Diseases

Daniel Emilio Dalledone Siqueira and
Ana Terezinha Guillaumon

Additional information is available at the end of the chapter

http://dx.doi.org/10.5772/intechopen.79232

Abstract

Renal Artery disease is one of the main causes of systemic arterial hypertension. Among its etiologies are atherosclerosis, fibromuscular dysplasia, Takayasu arteritis, among others. These diseases may evolve into stenosis, occlusion or aneurysms of the renal arteries. In the last decades, technological advances in both imaging diagnosis and treatment, have improved prognosis of patients, leading to earlier medical interventions. For the identification of renal vascular diseases, the adequate angiography technique as well as the capture of quality images are of utter importance. This chapter aims to address the main aspects of the renal artery diseases and their arteriographic findings.

Keywords: angiography, renal, atherosclerosis, nephropathy, fibromuscular dysplasia, renal aneurysm, Takayasu arteritis, kidney transplantation, diagnostic catheter

1. Introduction

The correct identification of renal vascular diseases by means of imaging techniques, among them the renal angiography, enables physicians to perform an appropriate morphological study and an efficient treatment [1]. Currently, new diagnostic and therapeutic methods have been developed and employed in the treatment of patients with renal vascular disease [2–4].

The present chapter is divided into three sections. The first section introduces the renal vascular anatomy, anatomical variations, renal angiography and its techniques. The second section examines the renal vascular diseases and their imaging findings. The third section presents other methods for the diagnosis of the renal vascular disease.

2. Renal angiographic morfology

2.1. Renal angiography

Renal angiography, despite the technological advances of the imaging methods, is still considered the final diagnostic method of the renal artery diseases. This method provides an anatomical visibility of the renal arteries when correct techniques are applied. Moreover, treatment decisions are made based on the lesion morphological aspects at arteriography. Another relevant aspect is that arteriography can provide images for immediate diagnostic and endovascular treatment during the procedure. A correct optimization of the arteriographic images provides an adequate assessment of the renal arteries, as well as of their segmental and subsegmental branches.

2.2. The renal angiography technique

Arterial access is obtained by inserting a 5F or 6F sheath into the femoral or brachial artery, using the modified Seldinger technique [5]. Ultrasound-guided arterial puncture can also be performed. A 5F catheter is positioned inside the aorta using the femoral or brachial artery access. Renal arteriography must start with the aortography, which aims to identify ostial stenosis of the renal arteries (**Figure 1**). Contrast material is injected manually or by means of an automatic injection pump, providing the sequence of images. The contrast volume, infusion speed, as well as the acquisition characteristics of the images, depend on each patient. Usual parameters include a 10–20 mL/K injection of contrast agent for 2 seconds. Images are usually registered for 3–5 seconds, about 1–2 images per second. However, this procedure may be extended for 3–5 additional seconds, depending on the images of interest, providing assessment of the intra-parenchymatous and venous arterial phases.

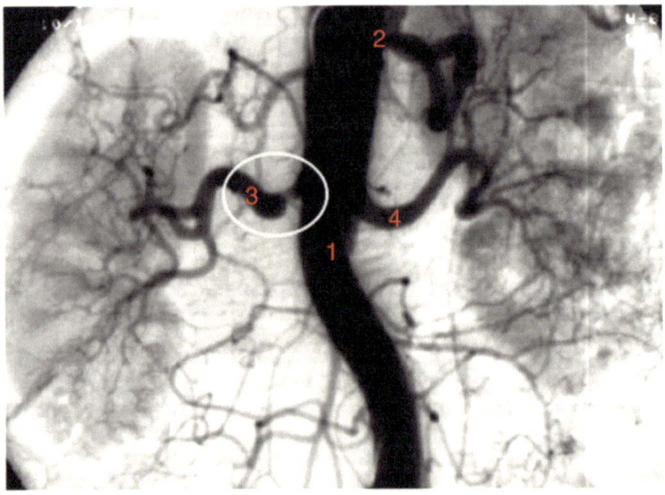

Figure 1. Aortography showing – (1) abdominal aorta; (2) superior mesenteric artery; (3) right renal artery, with atherosclerotic ostial stenosis; (4) left renal artery.

http://dx.doi.org/10.5772/intechopen.79232

Some technical details must be considered for the correct visibility of the renal parenchyma images. The side holes of the catheter must be positioned at the L1–L2 level. The correct positioning is necessary to prevent the contrast agent from filling the superior mesenteric artery, causing overlapping of images.

2.3. Selective catheterization of renal arteries

In some cases, depending on the quality of the images captured during aortography, it is necessary to perform selective catheterization of the renal arteries in order to better visualize the ostium and the distal branches, without the overlapping of the aorta and the branches. Selective catheterization must be performed with a preformed catheter such as Cobra, Renal Double Curved (RDC), Omni Selective, Simmons, among others. The renal intravenous contrast may be administered manually or with an injection pump. Volume of contrast agent is usually 3–6 mL/s, administered for 1–2 minutes.

Renal selective catheterization presents advantages in relation to aortography, as a smaller amount of contrast material is necessary to capture renal vessel images. Additionally, it offers the possibility to carry out a hemodynamic study of the stenosis by measuring the blood pressure before and after the lesion. Pressure gradient values cannot be obtained with other non-invasive diagnostic methods.

2.4. Registration methods of the angiographic images

Renal angiography may be performed by means of films or digital subtraction. In film-based angiography, X-ray images are recorded after the intravenous contrast injection. On the other hand, in digital subtraction angiography (DSA), the fluoroscopic images are produced in a sequence by means of an image intensifier (**Figure 2**). The captured images are electronically filed in digital format. The initial image, produced before contrast medium injection, is subtracted, generating a mask. All subsequent images are subtracted from this mask image, and only the contrast medium is visualized.

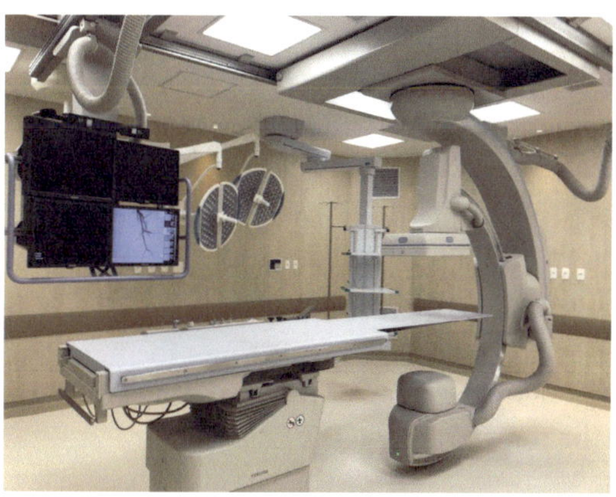

Figure 2. Hemodynamic room – School of Medical Sciences at Universidade Estadual de Campinas – UNICAMP.

2.5. Normal anatomy

The kidneys are a pair of retroperitoneal organs, located parallel to the spinal column, on the psoas major muscle, generally between L1 and L4 vertebrae level, in an orthostatic position. There may be a change in the position of both kidneys during the respiratory cycle, that is, during the inhalation and exhalation processes. This breathing variation may represent from 1 to 7 cm in the cranial-caudal position. In the supine position, the kidneys generally lie at the T12-L13 spinal segment level. The right kidney may be found slightly more caudal than the left kidney, due to the liver location. Both kidneys represent 0.4% of the total body weight and are approximately 11–13 cm long, the left kidney slightly longer than the right one.

Kidneys are related with the suprarenal gland, located above them, encapsulated by the renal fascia. Posteriorly situated are the diaphragm muscle, psoas major and quadratus lumborum muscles, the branches of the lumbar plexus, the 12 costal arch and the lateral edge of the erector spinae muscle. Anteriorly, they are covered by the peritoneum, the right kidney related to the posterior border of the liver and small intestine, whereas the left kidney is related to the stomach, spleen and small intestine.

At the medial border of the kidneys is a vertical fissure, called renal hilus, through which the renal vessels, nerves and ureter pass. Each kidney is structurally divided into cortex and medulla.

Renal arteries branch off the aorta, at the lateral side, right below the superior mesenteric artery, next to the L1–L2 vertebrae level [6, 7]. The right renal artery passes behind the inferior cava vein. Renal arteries are single in approximately 65% of the population and multiple in 35%. They are subdivided into segmental, interlobar and arcuate arteries.

Venous drainage takes place in the renal vessels, located anteriorly to the ipsilateral renal artery. Both veins drain into the inferior cava vein. Left renal vein is longer and receives tributary veins such as left gonadal vein, suprarenal vein, phrenic vein, among others. Right renal vein, on the other hand, is shorter, and generally does not receive tributaries.

2.6. Anatomical variations

Accessory renal arteries may be present in one or in both kidneys, corresponding to 25–35% of the general population [8]. Most accessory renal arteries supply the inferior pole of the kidney, arising from the suprarenal aorta to iliac arteries. Kidney anatomical alterations, such as ectopia, fusion and rotation, are associated with vascular alterations related to variations in origin and the number of renal arteries. In the horseshoe kidney, arterial irrigation is generally provided by three or more arteries, arising from the aorta or the iliac, or from both [9, 10].

Alterations in renal veins are usual. It is possible to observe the circumaortic left renal vein with retroaortic and pre-aortic segments, draining into the inferior cava vein. Additionally, multiple renal veins to the right, the retroaortic left renal vein and the right gonadal vein are observed, draining into the right renal vein [11, 12].

2.7. Renal collateral circulation

Renal arteries, despite being described as terminal branches of the abdominal aorta, present systems of collateralization, in cases of stenosis or occlusion. Intra-renal blood flow is provided by three collateral arterial systems, capsular, peripelvic and periureteral, which are supplied by lumbar arteries, abdominal aorta, internal iliac arteries, inferior adrenal arteries and other vessels [13].

In renal vein occlusion, blood flow is provided through ureteric, gonadal, adrenal, ascending lumbar and capsular veins [13].

3. Renal diseases and arteriographic morphology

3.1. Renal occlusive disease

Stenosis of the renal arteries may be defined as a multifactorial disease, of several etiologies, which affects the renal artery vasculature, at unilateral or bilateral level, determining various stenosis degrees, from its origin to the renal hilum [1, 14]. Clinically, it is presented as a renovascular hypertension and a renal ischemic disease and is associated with a higher cardiovascular risk and an increase in the mortality rate [15–18]. For research and treatment purposes, several authors suggest that renal artery stenosis is critical when it is greater than 60–70% [19].

The natural history of the renal atherosclerotic disease is still to be fully clarified. However, it is known that there is a progressive stenosis, associated with a decrease in the arterial flow, leading to an ultimate kidney failure, directly related to the stenosis degree of the renal artery [20, 21]. It is estimated that renovascular disease induces kidney failure in 5–15% of dialysis patients every year [22].

Prevalence of renal artery stenosis is controversial, as few population-based studies have been conducted to relate the disease to race, age and gender. Nevertheless, some research studies have demonstrated that renal artery stenosis affects 1–5% of patients with systemic arterial hypertension, representing the main cause of the secondary hypertension [1]. The disease is believed to account for 1% of the cases of mild to moderate hypertension and for 10–40% of the acute, severe and refractory hypertension cases [3]. Additionally, some population-based studies suggest that prevalence of the disease in patients older than 65 years of age is higher than 7% [1]. Random autopsy studies conducted in patients whose death was caused by other etiologies reveal that 4–50% of these patients presented renal arterial stenosis, 40% with no history of a systemic arterial hypertension [23].

Renal artery stenosis may present several etiologies, among them atherosclerosis, fibromuscular dysplasia (FMD) and Takayasu's arteritis (TAK) [24].

3.1.1. Renal occlusive disease: atherosclerosis

Atherosclerotic renal artery occlusion is more frequent and accounts for 70–80% of the cases. It is more prevalent in men, over 40 years of age, induces stenosis in the proximal segments of the renal arteries and is characterized by the presence of stenotic lesions at the proximal third of the renal arteries [25]. Morphologically, a renal artery atherosclerotic disease resembles eccentric atherosclerotic plaques, evolving towards the arterial lumen, with no precise aortic boundaries (**Figure 3**). It may affect the renal arteries at unilateral or bilateral levels, as well as the polar renal arteries, when they are present. Progression of the disease is observed in 50% of the cases, which may lead to bilateral stenosis, arterial occlusion, with or without renal infarction [20, 21].

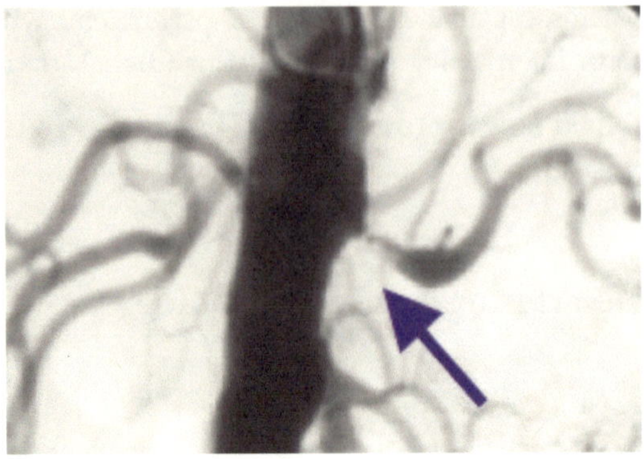

Figure 3. Atherosclerotic renal artery stenosis, located at the proximal third of the artery.

3.1.2. *Renal occlusive disease: fibromuscular dysplasia (FMD)*

Renal artery stenosis secondary to fibromuscular dysplasia accounts for 20–25% of the cases [26]. Fibromuscular dysplasia is a non-atherosclerotic and a non-inflammatory disease, which affects medium-sized arteries, rarely involving small-sized ones [27]. It is more prevalent in the Caucasian population, 15- to 50-year old women, affecting the more distal segments of the renal arteries and the intra-parenchymal segments. It may affect both renal arteries in 60% of the cases but is rarely observed in patients older than 60. Recent studies reveal that approximately 2% of renovascular hypertension are related to fibromuscular dysplasia [28].

Among the fibromuscular dysplasia types, the medial one is the most prevalent, the medial fibroplasia subtype accounting for 70–95% of dysplasia cases and 85% of the renovascular lesions [28]. Lesions predominantly affect the medial and distal third of the renal and polar arteries and their branches [26].

Arteriography may provide a high degree of diagnostic accuracy. The usual angiographic profile of medial fibroplasia resembles a string of bead (**Figure 4**). However, the gold standard procedure for the diagnosis of fibromuscular dysplasia is the histopathologic exam. The disease may evolve to renal artery stenosis or aneurysms and its diagnosis is usually an exam incidental finding, as fibromuscular dysplasia does not present alterations of inflammatory expressions such as hemosedimentation rate and C-reactive protein [29].

3.1.3. *Renal occlusive disease: Takayasu's arteritis (TAK)*

Takayasu's arteritis is a chronic, inflammatory and granulomatous disease, a vasculitis that affects large and middle-size arteries [30]. It is prevalent in women (80–90-% of the cases), starting between the age of 10 and 40 [31]. Initial symptoms are not specific, and include fever, general feeling of being unwell, weight loss and joint pains. There might be a vascular problem, which at the initial phase involves the thoracic and abdominal aorta and its main branches [32]. The inflammatory process induces the thickening of the arterial wall, leading to stenosis, occlusion or dilation of the affected arterial segments, at several stages [30]. In

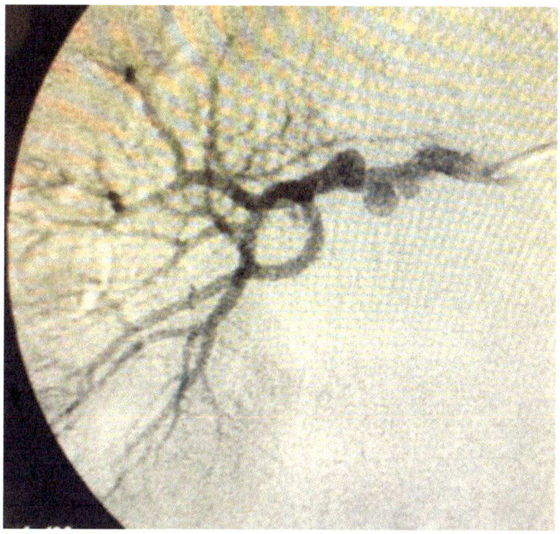

Figure 4. Morphological aspect of the fibromuscular dysplasia at selective angiography of the renal artery.

general, the clinical lab findings reveal elevated inflammatory markers, such as, C-reactive protein and hemosedimentation rate. Normocytic and normochromic anemia, and hypoalbuminemia reveal the chronic nature of the disease. Diagnostic criteria, defined by the American School of Rheumatology, include the development of signs and symptoms related to Takayasu's arteritis before the age of 40; claudication of the extremities, weakness; extremities discomfort and fatigue, more commonly in the upper limbs; decrease in the pulse rate amplitude in one or both brachial arteries; difference in the blood pressure of the upper limbs of at least 10 mmHg; murmur in one or both subclavian arteries; abdominal murmur; alterations in the arteriography: narrowing or occlusion of the aorta and /or its main branches or of the large proximal arteries in the lower and upper limbs, not caused by atherosclerosis or fibromuscular dysplasia. Three of the above criteria confirm the diagnosis, sensibility of 90.5% and specificity of 97.8%.

Renal arteries play an important role in the development of the disease in 50–60% of the cases [30–32]. It is clinically characterized by the renal occlusive disease, inducing renovascular hypertension or kidney failure. Treatment of patients affected by renovascular hypertension has been proven difficult. Generally, arteriography is required to confirm the diagnosis of the disease, characterized by its location in the proximal aorta and its branches (**Figure 5**). Nevertheless, due to the method limitation, angiography does not provide the identification of the arterial wall thickening. Other imaging methods for clinical investigation, such as computed angiotomography or angioresonance, are recommended.

3.2. Renal aneurysmal disease

The renal aneurysmal disease is uncommon and asymptomatic in most cases. Population-based studies show an incidence of 0.1% of the total population, representing 25% of the visceral aneurysm cases [33]. The actual prevalence is unknown, considering that it is a multifactorial disease and depends on the hereditary aspects of the studied population. Its

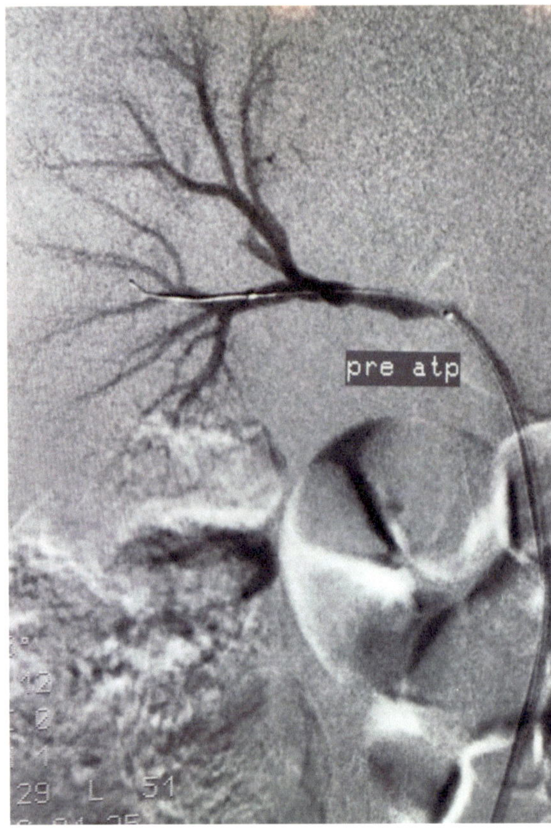

Figure 5. Aortography revealing renal artery occlusion induced by Takayasu's arteritis.

diagnosis usually represents an incidental finding during regular exams. It is more prevalent in women, in the right renal artery and rarely bilateral [34]. In most cases, they are solitary aneurysms, mostly saccular-shaped (**Figure 6**), accounting for 75% of the cases, but with some fusiform-shaped aneurysms as well, most often developed in the renal artery bifurcation, 90% of the cases extra-parenchymal and only 10% intra-parenchymal [35]. Among the various etiologies, the most prevalent is fibromuscular dysplasia. Other causes for the development of the renal aneurysmal disease include trauma, congenital diseases (Ehlers-Danlos syndrome and neurofibromatosis), inflammatory diseases, among others [35].

Renal arterial aneurysm presents low complication rates. Main complications are renovascular hypertension, renal artery thrombosis, renal infarction, distal embolization, formation of the arteriovenous fistula, dissection and rupture, the latter more common during pregnancy, mainly in the third trimester [36]. Maternal and fetal mortality rates associated with rupture during pregnancy are 55 and 85%, respectively [37].

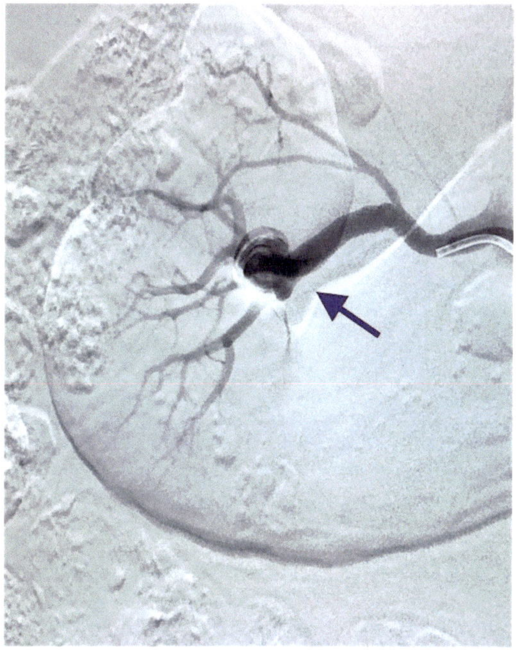

Figure 6. Selective arteriography of the renal artery revealing a saccular aneurysm.

Renal artery aneurysms may be classified according to their location: Type 1 in the main renal artery; Type 2 in the bifurcation and beginning of the segmental branches; Type 3 in the distal: intra-parenchymal artery.

Currently, several endovascular treatment methods have been developed to preserve renal function. Treatment indications reported by Henke et al., exhaustively revised, include: (1) renal artery aneurysms of over 1.0 cm in diameter, with a difficulty-to-control hypertension; (2) all renal artery aneurysms of over 2.0 cm in diameter; (3) most aneurysms of 1.5–2.0 cm in diameter. Some authors consider the possibility to treat all symptomatic renal artery aneurysms [35].

3.3. Kidney transplantation

Renal transplant represents a treatment option for the terminal renal disease. In this case, arteriography before and after the transplant provides better and thorough technical information.

Vascular complications are rare in renal transplants; however, they may lead to the loss of the transplanted kidney. Among the most common vascular complications are the renal artery stenosis (**Figure 7**), renal artery thrombosis, vascular lesions after biopsy, pseudoaneurysms and hematomas [38].

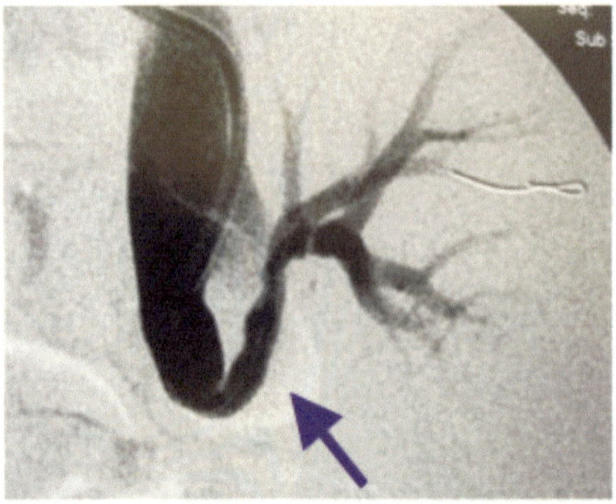

Figure 7. Selective arteriography of the transplanted kidney showing anastomotic stenosis.

4. Other diagnostic methods

The imaging study of the renal arteries may be performed by other diagnostic methods. In the last years, several imaging techniques have been developed in an attempt to precisely display the renal vascular anatomy, and obtain good quality of images, reproducibility and a lower rate of complications. Each method presents its advantages and disadvantages; however, in general, when compared, these exams are less invasive than renal angiography, considered a standard gold procedure [4].

4.1. Eco-Doppler

Eco-Doppler of renal arteries and veins has been widely used as an initial method in the investigation of vascular diseases. It combines the visualization of B-mode images and the measurement of blood flow velocities of renal arteries and veins as well as of specific indexes [39, 40]. Moreover, Eco-Doppler provides information related to renal anatomy, intra-renal vasculature, and kidney size.

4.2. Magnetic angioresonance

Magnetic angioresonance (MAR) has been largely used to complement Eco-Doppler investigation of the renal arteries. It is a less invasive method than angiography and provides images of a quality similar to that obtained at angiography. However, it requires neither arterial puncture nor nephrotoxic contrast medium to capture images [4].

The images generated by means of an electromagnetic field are compiled as multiple thin slices, adjacent and transversal. Additionally, tri-dimensional data from the images captured through magnetic angioresonance may be projected in multiple levels, providing better and thorough anatomic understanding of the images.

http://dx.doi.org/10.5772/intechopen.79232

4.3. Computed tomography (CT scan)

Computed angiotomography of the aorta and its branches is performed by administering an iodine-based contrast dye injection into a peripheral vein [4]. After the administration of the contrast material and the time necessary for each type of study, several sequential images are captured with a rotation platform. The images of the renal arteries are obtained at axial level, in thin slices, and then processed and reconstructed at several other levels with specific software programs, providing a tridimensional view (**Figure 8**).

The advantages of computed angiotomography include the possibility to measure the renal dimensions, the cortical thickness, the renal perfusion and vascular alterations in the aorta and its branches. On the other hand, the use of iodinated contrast media, known to be nephrotoxic, represents a risk factor mainly to nephropathic patients. The contrast volume used at angiotomography is larger than the one at digital subtraction angiography, 120–150 and 10–20 mL, respectively.

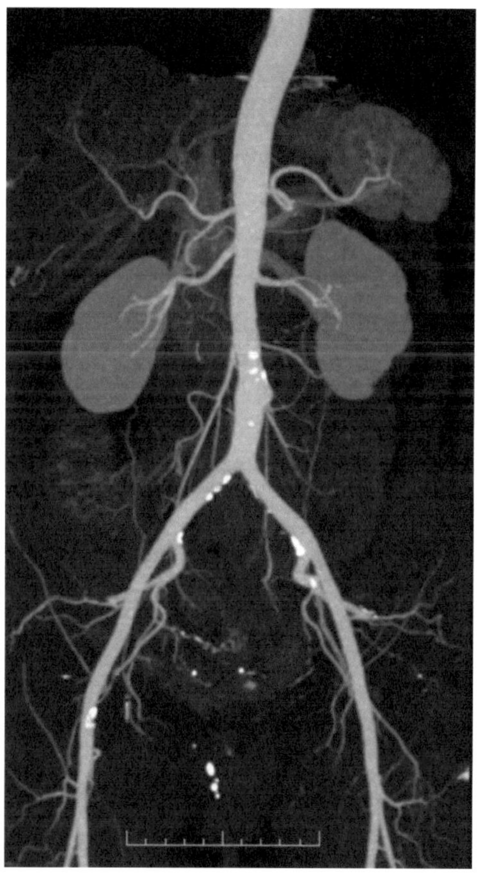

Figure 8. Computed angiotomography of the aorta and its branches, tridimensional view.

Author details

Daniel Emilio Dalledone Siqueira[1,2*] and Ana Terezinha Guillaumon[1,3,4]

*Address all correspondence to: siq_daniel@yahoo.com.br

1 School of Medical Sciences, UNICAMP, Brazil

2 Brazilian Society of Vascular Surgery – SBACV, Curitiba, Brazil

3 Vascular and Endovascular Surgery at the Hospital de Clínicas, UNICAMP, Brazil

4 Brazilian Society of Vascular Surgery – SBACV, Campinas, Brazil

References

[1] Cooper CJ, Murphy TP, Cutlip DE, Jamerson K, Henrich W, Reid DM, et al. Stenting and medical therapy for atherosclerotic renal-artery stenosis. The New England Journal of Medicine. 2014;**370**(1):13-22

[2] Rundback JH, Sacks D, Kent KC, Cooper C, Jones D, Murphy T, Rosenfield K, White C, Bettmann M, Cortell S, Puschett J, Clair D, Cole P. Guidelines for the reporting of renal artery revascularization in clinical trials. Circulation. 2002;**106**:1572-1585

[3] Safian RD, Textor SC. Renal artery stenosis. The New England Journal of Medicine. 2001;**344**:431-442

[4] Leiner T, de Haan MW, Nelemans PJ, van Engelshoven JMA, Vasbinder GBC. Contemporary imaging techniques for the diagnosis of renal artery stenosis. European Radiology. 2005; **15**:2219-2229

[5] Seldinger SI. Catheter replacement of the needle in percutaneous arteriography. Acta Radiologica. 1953;**39**:368-376

[6] Gabella G, editor. Cardiovascular system. In: Williams PL, Bannister LH, Berry MM, et al, editors. Gray's Anatomy. 38th ed. New York: Churchill Livingstone; 1995. p. 1557

[7] Dyson M, editor. In: Williams PL, Bannister LH, Berry MM, et al, editors. Gray's Anatomy, 38th ed. New York: Churchill Livingstone; 1995. p. 1826

[8] Rankin SC, Jan W, Koffman CG. Noninvasive imaging of living related kidney donors: Evaluation of CT angiography and gadolinium enhanced MR angiography. AJR. American Journal of Roentgenology. 2001;**177**:349

[9] Kaufman JA, Waltman AC, Rivitz SM, et al. Anatomical observations on the renal veins and inferior vena cava at magnetic resonance angiography. Cardiovascular and Interventional Radiology. 1995;**18**:153

[10] Hicks ME, Malden ES, Vesely TM, et al. Prospective anatomic study of the inferior vena cava and renal veins: Comparison of selective renal venography with cavography and relevance in filter placement. Journal of Vascular and Interventional Radiology. 1995;**6**:721

[11] Trigaux JP. Vandroogenbroek S, deWispelaere JF, et al: Congenital anomalies of the inferior vena cava and left renal vein: Evaluation with spiral CT. Journal of Vascular and Interventional Radiology. 1998;**9**:339

[12] Aljabri B, MacDonald PS, Satin R, et al. Incidence of major venous and renal anomalies relevant to aortoiliac surgery as demonstrated by computed tomography. Annals of Vascular Surgery. 2001;**15**:615

[13] Abrams HL, Cornell SH. Patterns of collateral flow in renal ischemia. Radiology. 1965;**84**:1001

[14] Guillaumon AT, Rocha EF, Medeiros CAF. Endovascular treatment of renal stenosis in solitary kidney. Journal of Vascular Surgery. 2008;**7**(2):99-105

[15] Minuz P, Patrignani P, Gaino S, Degan M, Menapace L, Tommasoli R, et al. Increased oxidative stress and platelet activation in patients with hypertension and renovascular disease. Circulation. 2002;**106**(22):2800-2805

[16] Kuller LH, Shemanski L, Psaty BM, Borhani NO, Gardin J, Haan MN, et al. Subclinical disease as an independent risk factor for cardiovascular disease. Circulation. 1995;**92**(4): 720-726

[17] O'Leary DH, Polak JF, Kronmal RA, Manolio TA, Burke GL, Wolfson SK. Carotid-artery intima and media thickness as a risk factor for myocardial infarction and stroke in older adults. The New England Journal of Medicine. 1999;**340**(1):14-122

[18] Newman AB, Shemanski L, Manolio TA, Cushman M, Mittelmark M, Polak JF, et al. Ankle-arm index as a predictor of cardiovascular disease and mortality in the cardiovascular health study. Arteriosclerosis, Thrombosis, and Vascular Biology. 1999;**19**(3):538-545

[19] Yu H, Zhang D, Haller S, et al. Determinants of renal function in patients with renal artery stenosis. Vascular Medicine. **2011**(5);16):331-338

[20] Guzman RP, Zierler RE, Isaacson JA, et al. Renal atrophy and arterial stenosis. A prospective study with duplex ultrasound. Hypertension. 1994;**23**(3):346-350

[21] Zierler RE, Bergelin RO, Davidson RC, et al. A prospective study of disease progression in patients with atherosclerotic renal artery stenosis. American Journal of Hypertension. 1996;**9**(11):1055-1061

[22] Watson PS, Hadjipetrou P, Cox SV, Piemonte TC, Eisenhauer AC. Effect of renal artery stenting on renal function and size in patients with atherosclerotic renovascular disease. Circulation. 2000;**102**(14):1671-1677

[23] Iglesias JI, Hamburguer RJ, Feldman L, Kaufman JS. The natural history of incidental renal artery stenosis in patients with aortoiliac vascular disease. The American Journal of Medicine. 2000;**109**(8):642-647

[24] Dean RH. Renovascular hypertension. Current Problems in Surgery. 1985;**22**(2):4-67

[25] Perkovic V, Thomson KR, Mitchell PJ, Gibson RN, Atkinson N, Field PL, et al. Treatment of renovascular disease with percutaneous stent insertion: Long-term outcomes. Australasian Radiology. 2001;**45**(4):438-443

[26] Persu A, Giavarini A, Touze E, Januszewicz A, Sapoval M, Azizi M, et al. European consensus on the diagnosis and management of fibromuscular dysplasia. Journal of Hypertension. 2014;**32**:1367-1378

[27] Olin JW, Gornik HL, Bacharach JM, Biller J, Fine LJ, Gray BH, et al. Fibromuscular dysplasia: State of the science and critical unanswered questions: A scientific statement from the American Heart Association. Circulation. 2014;**129**:1048-1078

[28] Olin JW, Scalove BA. Diagnosis, management and future developments of fibromuscular dysplasia. Journal of Vascular Surgery. 2011;**53**(3):826-836

[29] Poloskey SL, Olin JW, Mace P, Gornik HL. Fibromuscular dysplasia. Circulation. 2012;**125**(18):e636-e639

[30] Gotway MB, Araoz PA, Macedo TA, Stanson AW, Higgins CB, Ring EJ, et al. Imaging findings in Takayasu's arteritis. American Journal of Roentgenology. 2005;**184**:1945-1950

[31] Weaver FA, Kumar SR, Yellin AE, Anderson S, Hood DB, Rowe VL, et al. Renal revascularization in Takayasu arteritis-induced renal artery stenosis. Journal of Vascular Surgery. 2004;**39**:749-757

[32] Andrews J, Mason JC. Takayasu's arteritis-recent advances in imaging offer promise. Rheumatology (Oxford). 2007;**46**:6-15

[33] Stanley JC, Rhodes EL, Gewertz BL, et al. Renal artery aneurysms. Significance of macroaneurysms exclusive of dissections and fibrodysplastic mural dilations. Archives of Surgery. 1975;**110**:1327-1333

[34] Lumsden AB, Salam TA, Walton KG. Renal artery aneurysm: A report of 28 cases. Cardiovascular Surgery. 1996;**4**:185-189

[35] Henke PK, Cardneau JD, Welling THIII, et al. Renal artery aneurysms: A 35-year clinical experience with 252 aneurysms in 168 patients. Annals of Surgery. 2001;**234**:454-463

[36] Tham G, Ekelund L, Herrlin K, et al. Renal artery aneurysms. Natural history and prognosis. Annals of Surgery. 1983;**197**:348-352

[37] Cohen JR, Shamash FS. Ruptured renal artery aneurysms during pregnancy. Journal of Vascular Surgery. 1986;**6**:51-59

[38] Bruno S, Remuzzi G, Ruggenenti P. Transplant renal artery stenosis. Journal of the American Society of Nephrology. 2004;**15**:134-141

[39] De Bruyne B, Manoharan G, Pijls NHJ, Verhamme K, Madaric J, Bartunek J, Vanderheyden M, Heyndrickx GR. Assessment of renal artery stenosis severity by pressure gradient measurement. Journal of the American College of Cardiology. 2006;**48**:1851-1855

[40] Strandness DE Jr. Duplex imaging for the detection of renal artery stenosis. American Journal of Kidney Diseases. 1994;**24**:674-678

Section 4

Interventions in Structural Heart Diseases

Chapter 7

Transcatheter Closure of Congenital VSDs: Tips and Tricks

Behzad Alizadeh

Additional information is available at the end of the chapter

http://dx.doi.org/10.5772/intechopen.83641

Abstract

Nowadays transcatheter device closure of ventricular septal defects (VSDs) is an attractive and feasible alternative to surgical closure of congenital VSDs. Isolated congenital VSDs constitute the most common form of congenital heart disease (CHD) in infants and children and account for 20–30% of all types of cardiac malformations. Most of the VSDs are located in the membranous portion of the ventricular septum (perimembranous VSDs). There are also less common types of VSDs located in the muscular portion (muscular VSDs), below the pulmonary valve (subpulmonary or supracristal VSDs), and near the junction of the tricuspid and mitral valves (inlet type VSDs). Indications for closure of VSDs include a hemodynamically significant left to right shunt and prevention of long-term complications, including pulmonary hypertension, progressive ventricular dilatation, aortic insufficiency, double-chambered right ventricle, and endocarditis. In this chapter, we review the technical details for achieving a successful procedure, as well as some tips and tricks on using off-label devices during transcatheter approach in VSD closure.

Keywords: congenital VSD, transcatheter device closure

1. Introduction

Ventricular septal defect (VSD) is the most common congenital heart defect and accounts for approximately 20% of all forms of congenital heart disease as an isolated lesion with incidence increasing up to 40% in case of multiple congenital heart defects [1]. Perimembranous VSDs are the most common form (70%), and muscular (15–20%) and sub arterial (5%) are less common (**Figure 1**). The size of the defect determines the size of the left to right shunt, which affects the hemodynamic state from negligible to cardiac failure and mild to severe

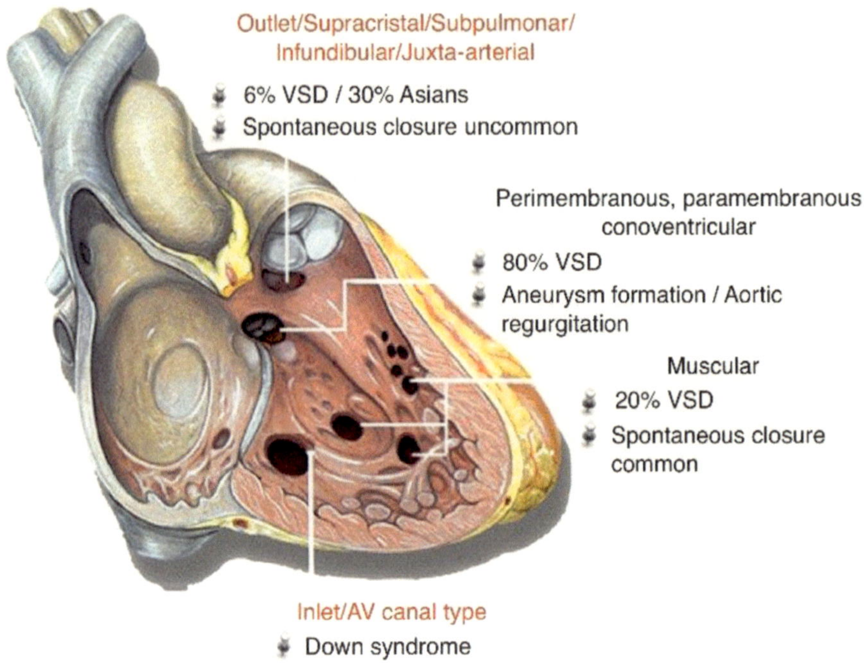

Figure 1. Prevalence of different forms of VSDs (picture courtesy: Patrick J Lynch; C. Carl Jaffe Yale University).

pulmonary hypertension. Although most of the larger defects persist through adulthood, some smaller defects have a high likelihood of spontaneous closure. There are some long-term complications of VSDs including prolapse of aortic cusps with regurgitation, infective endocarditis, arrhythmias, and pulmonary hypertension, which may lead to pulmonary vascular obstructive disease or Eisenmenger syndrome.

Traditionally, closure of ventricular septal defects (VSDs) has been a surgical procedure for over 50 years with a low operative mortality and postoperative morbidity. However, in 1988, Lock et al. [2] reported the results of transcatheter VSD closure using the Rashkind double umbrella device in six patients with congenital and acquired VSDs. Transcatheter closure of VSD as an alternative to surgery has now gained increasing acceptance due to a comparable success rate and low risk of complications. This approach has several advantages, such as avoidance of sternotomy and cardiopulmonary bypass, with less pain and no scar and shorter hospital stay, as well. There are also some disadvantages like the need for X-ray and contrast media injections.

Although surgical treatment remains the standard approach for VSDs, percutaneous device closure has brought hope to be a safe and effective treatment with a high rate of success.

2. Historical aspects

Transcatheter closure of ventricular septal defects was first described by Rashkind when he used a single-disc device to perform this in dogs.

Lock et al. used Rashkind double disc PDA umbrella in human subsequently. Six of the seven devices were implanted successfully in his series, while the seventh embolized into the pulmonary artery. Goldstein used clamshell occluder to close the VSDs. Gianturco coils, Amplatzer membranous and muscular devices, buttoned device, wireless devices (detachable steel coils, detachable balloon, and transcatheter patch), cardioSEAL/STARFlex devices, Nit-occlud (Nickel-Titanium Spiral Coil), and Amplatzer Duct Occluder I and Amplatzer Duct Occluder II devices were used for transcatheter occlusion of VSDs subsequently.

Postmyocardial infarction VSDs were also closed percutaneously using Rashkind double disc PDA umbrella, clamshell, CardioSEAL or STARFlex, Amplatzer septal occluder, Amplatzer duct occluder, and Amplatzer post-infarct muscular VSD (PIMVSD) successfully.

Amplatzer muscular VSD and PIMVSD occluders, Qwik-Load and STARFlex Septal Occlusion System, and CardioSEAL Septal Occlusion System are now approved by FDA, but there are multiple devices that have been used to close VSDs so far, which include VSD Le Coils, Muscular and Membranous VSD devices of Occlutech Co., and many Chinese symmetrical and Asymmetrical VSD occluders and the Amplatzer Duct occluder with Duct Occluder II (St. Jude Medical, Inc.) as well. The use of the Chinese devices is most commonly reported from China itself. Although the Amplatzer membranous VSD occluder was found useful, development of heart block precipitated its removal from clinical trials in the USA. Other devices are in clinical trials in either the USA or abroad [1].

3. Indications

Different patients with VSDs may present with different scenarios. Most muscular VSDs and a few perimembranous type may close spontaneously in early month of life. Some large unrestrictive VSDs may cause heart failure and failure to thrive in small babies. These infants need a large device for interventional closure, which makes the procedure difficult and unsafe. So this group of patient often refers to surgeons.

Although closure of VSDs in patients with aortic valve prolapse or AI remains controversial and most of this patients with trivial AI are now referred to surgeons, Le VSD Coil (pfm medical ag, Koln, Germany) occluder has recently used in such condition with good results [2].

VSDs are considered eligible for transcatheter device closure in the presence of one or more of the following indications:

- Evidence of heart failure not controlled by medical therapy
- Pulmonary to systemic blood flow ratio greater than 1.5 ($Qp/Qs > 1.5$)
- Evidence of left heart volume over load
- History of previous endocarditis

3.1. Contraindications

- body weight less than 6 kg
- pulmonary vascular resistance index greater than 7 WU/m^2, unresponsive to oxygen

- PMVSD extending to the inlet
- the presence of additional lesions requiring surgical intervention (ToF)
- when parents prefer surgical intervention.

Pulmonary hypertension is defined as a mean pulmonary artery pressure of 20 mm Hg or greater based on the original natural history studies [3].

There are some other considerations like distance from the edge of the VSD to the semilunar valves:

- <2 mm—for the Amplatzer membranous VSD occlude
- <4 mm—for the Nit-Occlud VSD

4. Preprocedure assessment

Echocardiography can provide valuable information on the number, the location, the size, and the relationship of the VSD to the adjacent structures. In addition, transesophageal and 3D-echocardiography are now widely available and may provide additional information of unusual VSDs.

5. Technique

5.1. General considerations

Compared to patent ductus and atrial septal defect closure, VSD closure is considerably more complicated. It is thus important to recognize that this procedure should only be undertaken in well-equipped units with sufficient skill, knowledge, and surgical backup.

- Anesthesia: the procedure may be performed under general anesthesia, although sedation can be used.
- Imaging: most of the centers use continuous transesophageal echocardiography (TEE), but skilled echo cardiographers may use transthoracic echo during the procedure.
- Catheterization: a comprehensive evaluation should be done during angiography to obtain different views at multiple angles of the VSD and a complete study for valvular function and regurgitation as well.
- Access: although in some certain muscular VSDs, the right internal jugular vein access may be used, and femoral artery and vein are usually gained as the main access. Alternatively, in small patients who making an arteriovenous circuit may cause hemodynamic instability when long stiff sheath is placed across the tricuspid valve, a hybrid approach can be used.

http://dx.doi.org/10.5772/intechopen.83641

In some selected older children with some difficulties, the VSD may be approached retrogradely from the femoral artery. Activated clotting time is maintained above 200 seconds throughout the procedure.

- Device selection: the device is usually selected 1–2 mm larger than the maximal diameter of the defect as assessed by TEE and angiography. Balloon sizing is hardly ever used, since the inter-ventricular septum is regarded to be a nonstretchable structure. There are some other important considerations in device selection but paying attention to the location, shape, morphology, and length and thickness of the edges of defect are of the most important factors (**Figures 2** and **3**).

- Crossing the VSD: normally, the VSD is crossed from the left ventricle using a Judkins right coronary artery catheter, but a variety of tip angled catheters can be used based on the defect location and shape like Bern, Cobra or a cutoff Pigtail. An exchange guidewire like Terumo or Noodle wire is then placed into the left or right pulmonary artery via the VSD crossed catheter (**Figure 4B**).

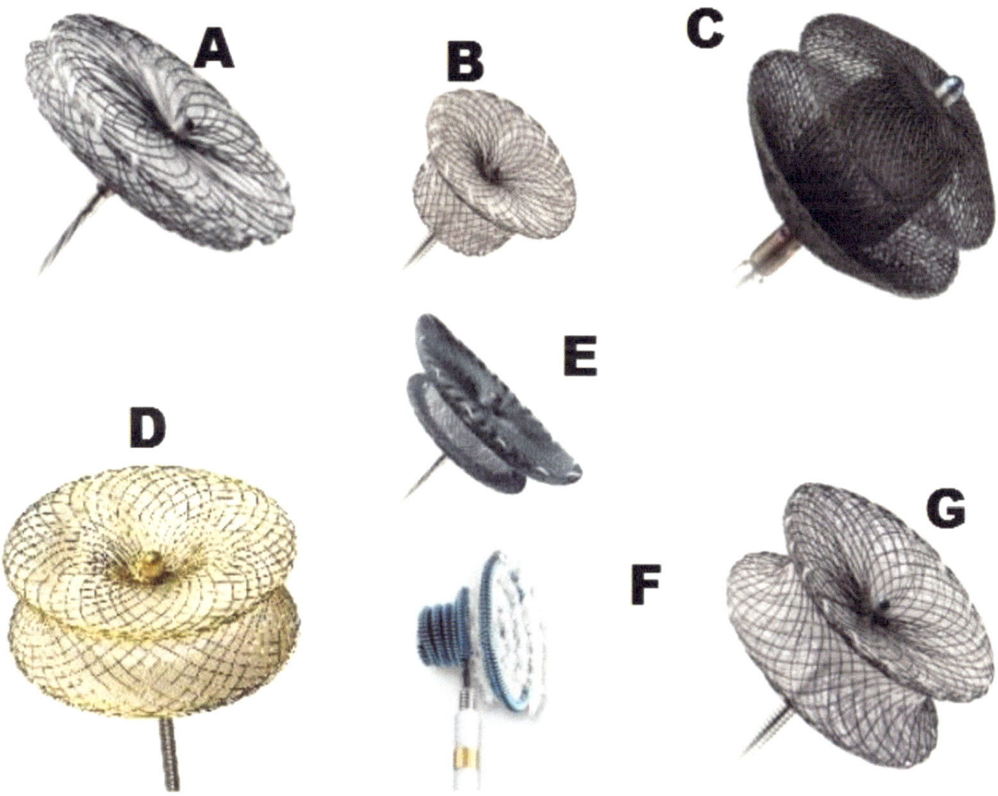

Figure 2. (A) Amplatzer membranous VSD device, (B and C) Amplatzer Duct Occluder and Amplatzer Duct Occluder II devices. (D and G) Amplatzer and Occlutech muscular VSD device. (F) Nit-Occlud (Nickel-Titanium Spiral Coil) and (E) asymmetric membranous VSD device were used for transcatheter occlusion of VSDs.

- Arteriovenous guide wire loop: to make an arteriovenous wire loop, the guide wire is then snared and pulled out via the right femoral vein. A delivery sheath will be then advanced via the femoral vein access into right ventricle into the aorta carefully. Undue tension on the arteriovenous loop and VSD may cause rhythm disturbances. To avoid direct contact of the guide wire with the VSD when crossed by the sheath, a "kissing catheter technique" should be used. The delivery sheath is then positioned to a suitable position in the left ventricle or descending aorta (**Figure 4C,D**).
- The device: the proper size and suitable shape device is then screwed to the tip of the delivery cable and advanced to the cavity of left ventricle or descending aorta via the long sheet with special care to avoid the occurrence air embolism. The LV disc is first deployed within the LV chamber or descending aorta and gently pulled back to the intra-ventricular VSD under echo or angiographic guidance. The waist of the device and right ventricular disc are then deployed, respectively. Careful attention should be paid to good positioning and stability of the device and any potential compromising of the adjusting structures. In the case of any impingent of valves or other structures, the device can still be recaptured into the sheath and repositioned gently. Once proper positioning has been achieved, the device may be released by unscrewing it counter clockwise using the pin vice. After release, confirmation of correct positioning should be established using TEE or TTE and angiography (**Figures 4F–I** and **5**).

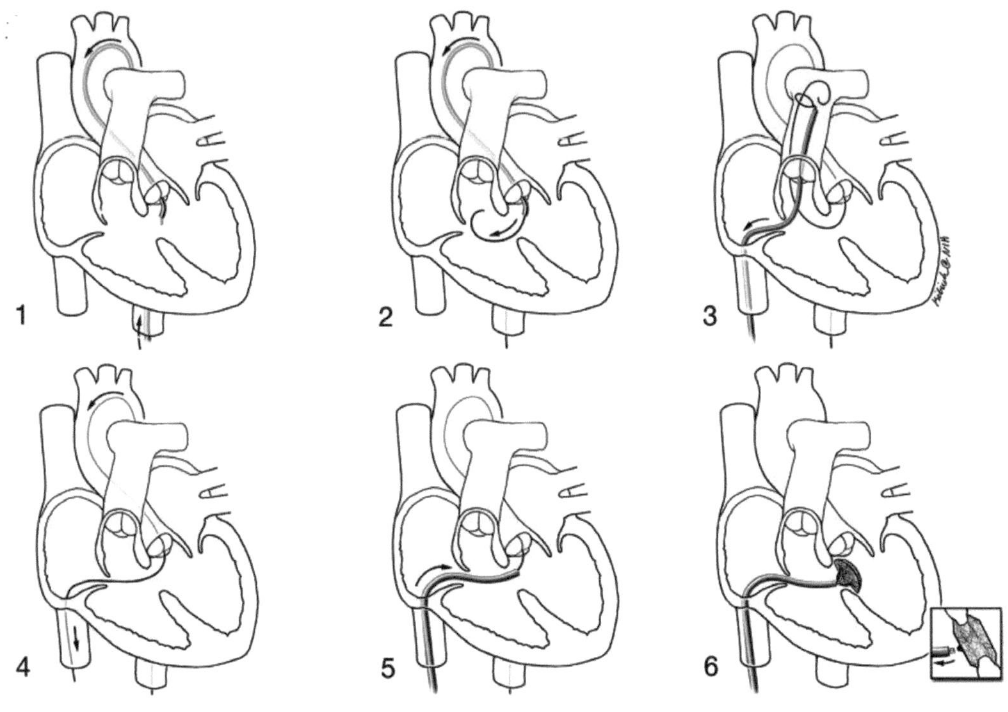

Figure 3. Schematic depictions of conventional technique. 1—Transaortic access into LV chamber retrogradely. 2—Crossing a guide wire from LV to RV chamber retrogradely. 3—Snaring the trans-aortic guide wire from the pulmonary artery. 4—Making an arteriovenous loop to provide a way to deliver the VSD delivery sheath. 5—The delivery sheath is advanced antegradely across the VSD. 6—The device is fixed in position and released. (Courtesy of Lydia Kibiuk, NIH Medical Arts and Photography Branch).

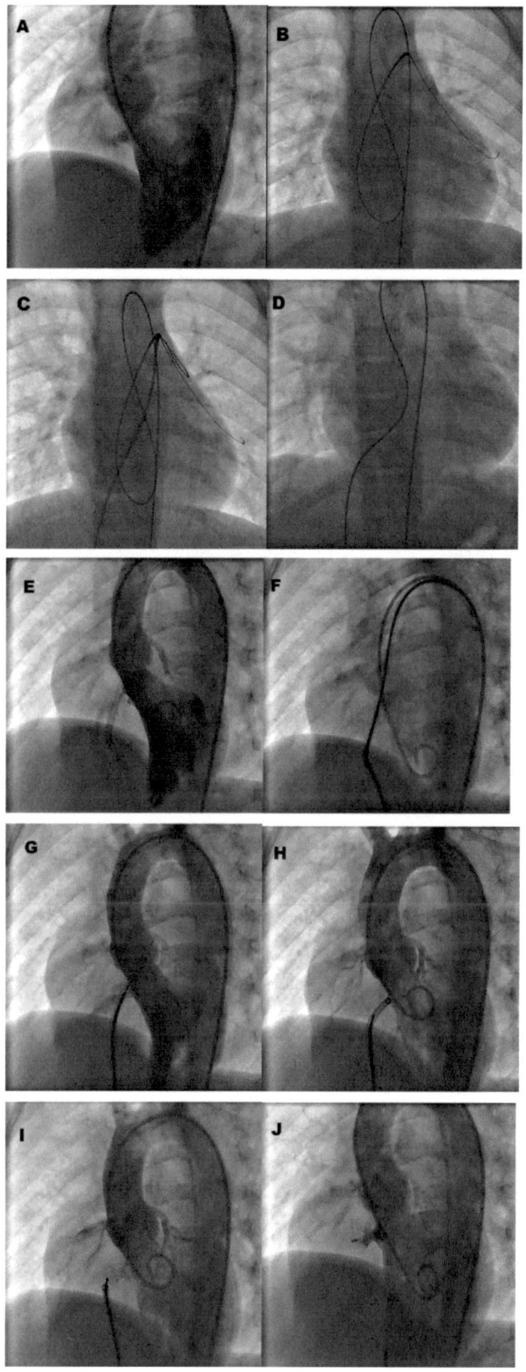

Figure 4. Stepwise percutaneous VSD closure technique using CaridoFix Muscular VSD Occluder. (A) Small upper muscular VSD. (B) Crossing the VSD and putting the wire in pulmonary artery. (C) Snaring the pulmonary wire via venous access. (D) Making the AV loop from arterial and venous access. (E) Crossing the VSD by long sheet and into the descending aorta. (F) Releasing the first disc of the device. (G) Pulling back the device. (H) Fixing the device to the septum. (I) Releasing the second disc of the device. (J) Complete deploying and releasing of the device.

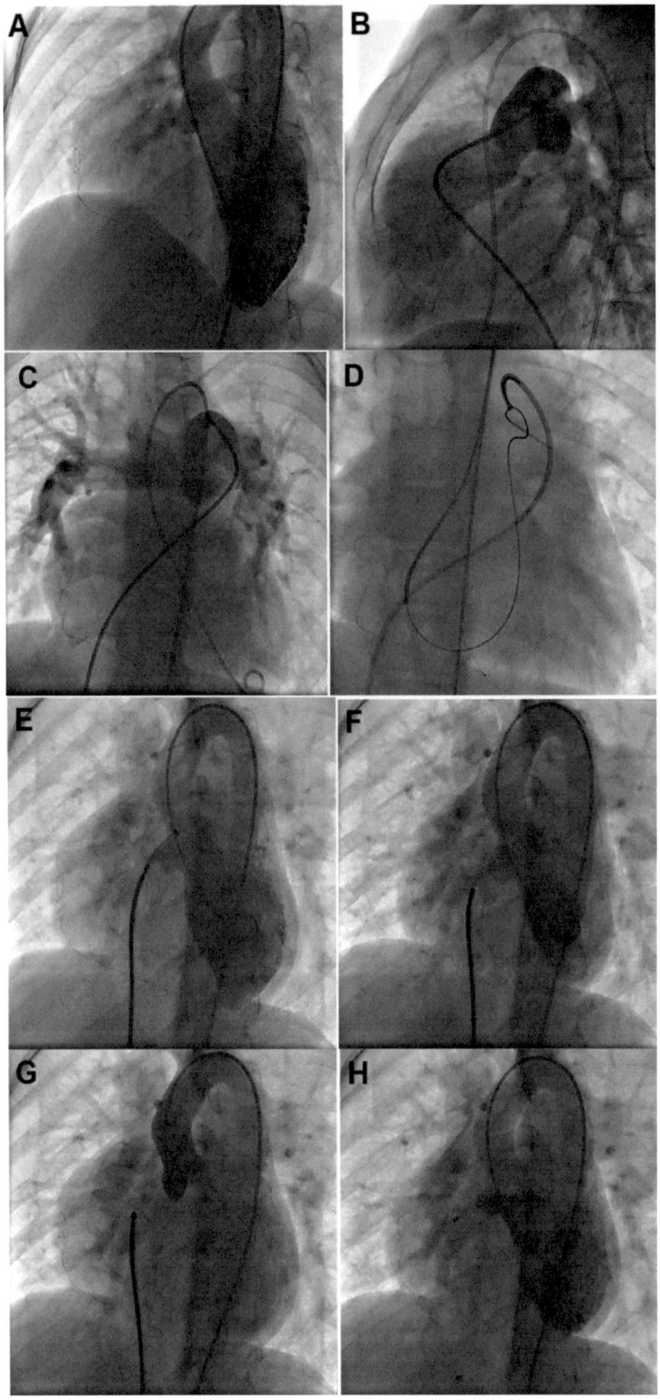

Figure 5. Post operation residual VSD closure technique in a patient with TOF using Occutech Duct Occluder. (A) Small residual VSD around the patch. (B) Main pulmonary injection showing free PI (lateral view). (C) Main pulmonary injection showing free PI (AP view). (D) Snaring the pulmonary wire via venous access making the AV loop. (E) Crossing the VSD into the ascending aorta and releasing the first disc of the device. (F) Pulling back the device and fixing the device to the septum. (G) Aortic root injection, checking the device position and probable AI. (H) Releasing the device.

http://dx.doi.org/10.5772/intechopen.83641

- Early postprocedure care: three doses of an antibiotic should be given to the patient within the 24 hours of observation with ECG monitoring. Endocarditis prophylaxis and a low dose of an anti-platelet agent like aspirin are recommended for 6 months [4].

5.2. Complications

The complications may occur immediately after the procedure or late during the follow up.

Device embolization: both systemic and right heart embolization of the device may occur and have been reported in up to 2% of cases. Continues TEE or intermittent TTE during the procedure and especially before the releasing of the device is crucial and very helpful. Operators should be familiar with retrieval techniques, and all necessary equipment for retrieval should be available. Surgical backup is also considered essential [5].

Dysrhythmias: during catheter and device manipulation, temporary dysrhythmias, usually ventricular, are common. Right bundle branch block occurred in only 6% of patients (5) compared to up to 64% of reported surgical series. Complete atrioventricular block (cAVB) is also a potential complication of transcatheter or surgical VSD closure. The reported cases of cAVB are mostly attributed to direct compression trauma, the pressure of radial forces (shape memory of the device), clamping forces, inflammatory processes, and/or the use of oversized devices [6].

Valvular malfunction: the device may influence function of any of the adjacent valves, but especially with the membranous device, aortic and tricuspid regurgitation should actively be looked for with TTE or TEE prior to release of the device.

Hemolysis: blood scape through a small residual shunt after VSD device closure may lead to hemolysis. To be aware of this potential complication especially when there is a residual shunt is very important. Checking the patient's urine color change in early hours after the procedure is a simple way to detect the hemolysis. Some form of little hemolysis may be self-limited and could be managed conservatively but in the form of massive hemolysis blood transfusion and surgical removal of the device should be considered.

Author details

Behzad Alizadeh

Address all correspondence to: behalizadeh@yahoo.com

Pediatric and Congenital Cardiology Department, Mashhad University of Medical Sciences, Imam Reza University Hospital, Mashhad, Iran

References

[1] Balzer D. Current status of percutaneous closure of ventricular septal defects. Pediatrics and Therapeutics. 2012;**2**:112

[2] Lock JE, Block PC, McKay RG, Baim DS, Keane JF. Transcatheter closure of ventricular septal defects. Circulation. 1988;**78**:361-368

[3] Weidman WH, Blount SG Jr, Dushane JW, Gersony WM, Hayes CJ, Nadas AS. Clinical course in ventricular septal defect. Circulation. 1977;**56**(1 Suppl):I56

[4] Brown SC, Bruwer AD, Smit FE. Percutaneous closure of ventricular septal defects in childhood. SA Heart Journal. 2017;**4**(1):26-31

[5] Sanz AP, Álvarez-Fuente M, Centella T, del Cerro MJ. Early complete atrioventricular block after percutaneous closure of a perimembranous ventricular septal defect with a Nit-Occlud (®) Lê VSD coil. Progress in Pediatric Cardiology. 2018;**49**:81-83

[6] Ratnayaka K, Raman VK, Faranesh AZ, Sonmez M, Kim JH, Gutiérrez LF, et al. Antegrade percutaneous closure of membranous ventricular septal defect using X-ray fused with magnetic resonance imaging. JACC: Cardiovascular Interventions. 2009;**2**(3):224-230

Section 5

Computed Tomography Angiography in Coronary and Periferal Arterial Diseases

Chapter 8

Computer-Aided Detection, Pulmonary Embolism, Computerized Tomography Pulmonary Angiography: Current Status

Abdel-Razzak M. Al-hinnawi

Additional information is available at the end of the chapter

http://dx.doi.org/10.5772/intechopen.79339

Abstract

Angiography (mostly computed tomography, but in some cases, conventional) is still the gold diagnostic standard in the clinical diagnosis of pulmonary embolism (PE). Computer-aided detection (CAD) is software that alerts radiologists the presence of PE during computerized tomography pulmonary angiography (CTPA) examinations. Interpreting CTPA scans with the aid of commercially available CTPA-CAD has improved the detectability of PE patients. This chapter aims to complete the scope of this book by explaining the clinical evidences of PE, the CTPA technology, the role of CTPA-CAD software in improving the diagnostic abilities of CTPA and the role of conventional pulmonary angiography in daily clinical practice. The reader will be introduced to the performance of diagnosing PE with or without the aid of CTPA-CAD algorithms. Differences among CTPA-CAD's output will be compared and tabled according to "per patient," "per clot," "first reader," and "second reader" basis. This includes, but not limited to, the CTPA-CAD's sensitivity and specificity in comparison to human observer performance (i.e., radiologist). These topics cover the *current status* practice at the pulmonary angiography clinic.

Keywords: computer-aided detection, computerized tomography pulmonary angiography, pulmonary embolism, digital image processing, conventional pulmonary angiography

1. Introduction

Computer sciences have reached medicine [1]. This includes developing algorithms to participate in the clinical interpretation of medical images acquired from various medical imaging systems [2, 3]. These algorithms are categorized into two main groups. They are the computer-aided detection (CAD) and the computer-aided diagnosis (CADx) [2, 3]. Both of them employ principles of digital image processing (DIP).

Pulmonary embolism (PE) is the partial or complete blockage of one or some of pulmonary arteries; it is a life threatening disease with a challenging diagnosis [4]. In Europe and the USA, it leads to high incidence of mortality, morbidity, and hospitalization [4, 5]. Internationally, PE is expected to become the third leading cause of death by 2030 according to clinical projections on disease mortality [6]. Computerized tomography pulmonary angiography (CTPA) has become the first-line imaging examination to detect the occurrence of PE [4, 7–9]. Clinical trials of CTPA examination, without the aid of CAD, reported that the sensitivity and specificity CTPA scan may not reach 100% [8, 10]. This indicates that misdiagnoses, which are a prospective health burden and potential life threatening, may occur.

This chapter describes the current state of PE diagnosis in CTPA clinic, with and without the use of CAD algorithms. The chapter is divided into three main sections. Section 2 presents all clinical evidences about the PE as a disease that threaten lives. This covers the PE epidemiology, incidence rate, characterizations, load scores, diagnosis, and treatment. Section 3 is dedicated to explain the CTPA physics and technology, image appearance, PE radiographic features, clinical trials, and common artifacts. Section 4 explains the art of computer-assisted detection and its applications in diagnosing PE. This demonstrates the role of CAD software in improving the PE diagnosis. In general, this chapter provides the up-to-date knowledge of PE diagnosis in angiography clinics.

2. Pulmonary embolism

2.1. Definition

Pulmonary embolism (PE) occurs when a blood clot, also known as a thrombus or embolus, arrives to pulmonary arteries. The source of thrombus is likely to be large veins of the lower extremity before it migrates through venous system to reach first the right heart chambers and later the lungs (**Figure 1**). Once a clot arrives to pulmonary arterial tree, it travels in the arteries of the lung until it blockades vessel/s that is/are too narrow to continue further. Thus, PE happens (**Figure 1**) leading to pulmonary blood flow shortage. Consequently, this condition associates with rise in the artery pressure due to the increased resistance to the bloodstream, shortness of breath, chest pain, and breathing difficulties; it can also lead to infarct or decrease in cardiac output, which in turn can cause hemodynamic disturbances, heart failure or even death [4, 5, 11, 12]. The common risk factors for PE are immobility or inactivity, hypertension, surgery or trauma, cigarette smoking, obesity, heart failure, cancer, chronic obstructive lung disease, hormone therapy, pregnancy, and advanced age and family members with thrombosis or embolism [4, 5, 12].

2.2. Incidence

Clinical surveys showed that the PE exhibits the highest incidence of mortality, morbidity, and hospitalization [4, 5, 13, 14]. The incidence of PE vary from one country to other but this

http://dx.doi.org/10.5772/intechopen.79339

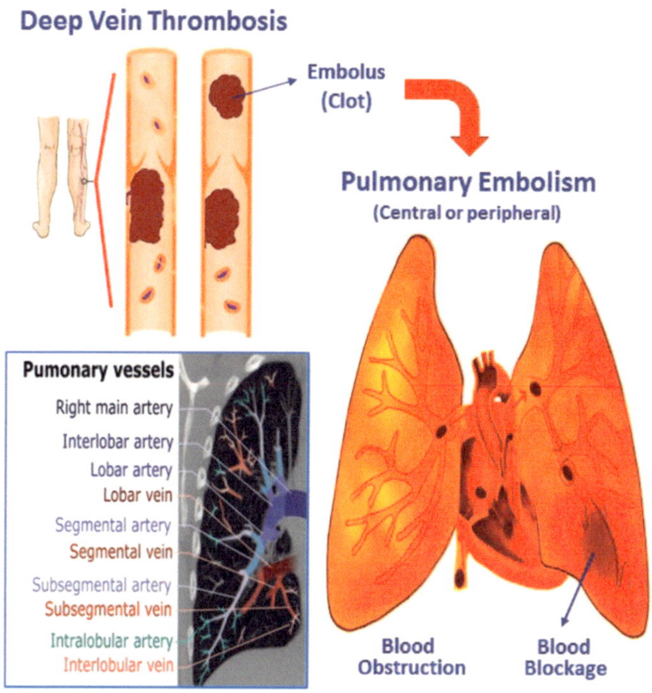

Figure 1. Pulmonary embolism pathophysiology.

variation is likely attributed to the type and accuracy of the diagnostic procedure rather than the actual incidence of the disease itself [6, 15–18]. Annually, there are 430,000 and 300,000 to 600,000 PE conditions in Europe and the USA, respectively [15, 16]. Globally, the clinical projections of mortality estimate that the incidence of PE will be the third major cause of death in year 2030 [6]. In Europe and the USA, autopsy investigations on hospitalized patients showed a PE prevalence from 60 to 70% [4, 5]. Therefore, the precise detection and diagnosis are highly desirable [4, 5].

2.3. Characterization

Embolus is characterized as central or peripheral, based on the site of the affected blood vessel branch [4]. Central vascular regions include the left and right main pulmonary arteries (PA), the right and left interlobar arteries, the right and left lobar arteries, and right and left lobar veins (**Figure 1**). Peripheral vascular regions include the remaining blood vessels in the upper, middle, and lower lobes of the right lung; and the upper and lower lobes in the left lung. This includes all the segmental, subsegmental, and intralobular arteries and veins including the culmen and the lingual (**Figure 1**).

Once a thrombus has been identified in the PA, it is further characterized as acute or chronic, as illustrated in **Figure 2** [4]. In some cases, there is doubt between those two classes, depending on diagnosis procedure and experience of the observer. A clot in PA is usually considered as being "acute" if it is located centrally within the vascular lumen. This may lead to vessel dilation. However, a clot in PA is characterized as "chronic" when it appears contiguous to

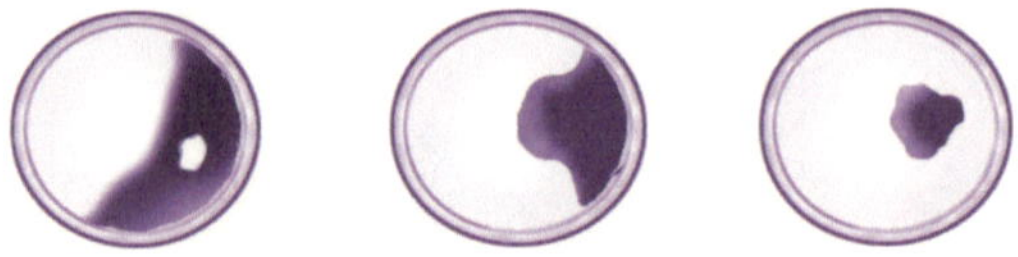

Figure 2. Illustration of acute and chronic PE.

the vessel wall substantially reducing the arterial diameter. A clot that exhibits caves or canals within itself is also considered as "chronic."

2.4. Load scores

Several scoring systems have been introduced to measure the severity of the PE clinic. For central PE, physicians utilize the Walsh, Miller, Qanadli, or Mastora score. While for peripheral PE, they use Marder, Arnesen, Mewissen (American Venous Registry), Porter, Ouriel, or Bjorgell scores. They are well summarized by Ghaye et al. [19, 20]. All these scores depend on the number of clots, location, and the percentage of obstruction. They all verified appropriate for assessing the severity of PE and treatment effectiveness, but are not much used in angiography clinics due to time it takes to manually assess them.

2.5. Diagnosis

Diagnosing PE remains a challenge to physicians because the symptoms are unspecific and may not be present in all patients. The PE symptoms and risk factors (Section 2.1) are used to determine the probability of PE. Although biomarkers and laboratory tests are crucial to estimate the probability of PE, such as the electrocardiogram (ECG) and the measurement of percentage of cross-linked fibrin in the blood (D-dimer), the diagnostic decision is always based on radiographic findings from medical imaging procedures [4]. Different medical imaging techniques exist to "rule in" or "rule out" the presence of the PE. Each technique exhibits its strength and weakness and a shift toward the computerized tomography (CT) has been approved.

A planner chest X-ray remains the first imaging step because it can rule out the conditions that mimic PE (e.g., a pneumothorax can cause chest pain similar to pain caused by acute PE), but it cannot exclude PE. Another X-ray imaging test is the lower extremity venous angiography, in which contrast media is injected via a foot vein, and several X-ray projections contrast-filled leg veins are taken [4]. The leg veins are "opacified" with contrast media, indicating the site of blood flow obstruction due to thrombosis. In both diagnosis situations, that is venous thrombosis is ruled in or out, further medical imaging tests are required to assess the decision of PE, which implies burden and probably additional radiation dose to patient.

Nuclear medicine techniques (e.g., pulmonary ventilation perfusion scintigraphy) permit the visualization of the distribution of a radioactive substance (i.e., radiopharmaceutical) through planner gamma camera or single photon emission computerized tomography (SPECT) [21, 22]. In this technique, after the administration of gamma ray isotope tracer, the observation of airways and pulmonary blood vessels activity is made, hence the name, ventilation/perfusion

(V/Q) scan. This scan remained as the traditional preferred imaging technique before the shift toward CT [4]. A mismatch of ventilated but not perfused lung tissue was considered as indicator for pulmonary embolism. Thus, it is indirect detection of an embolus by looking at the effects of an occlusion. A normal perfusion scan securely excluded pulmonary embolism, but was found in a minority of the patients that are suspected of PE, and thus, often further testing was needed [4]. The advantages of V/Q scan are that it is not invasive and less irradiant than CT, and may be more suitable for patients that are allergic to iodinated agents (CT). Its disadvantage is that the obtained image determines only regions of the lungs that are not correctly vascularized, nonobstructing "small" clots remaining invisible [4]. Moreover, the duration of the exam is in the order of 20 min, which is slower than other modalities. Several reports showed that the CT scan outweigh the V/Q scan by performing both lower rate of false-negative scans and lower number of "indeterminate scans" not yielding a definite diagnosis [4, 22].

The sequence of chest X-ray projections during the administration of contrast agent directly into the target vessels, also called as pulmonary angiography, is a reliable test for diagnosing PE. In this imaging scan, a catheter is inserted into a femoral vein and navigated through the heart toward the pulmonary arteries. Amounts of contrast media is injected several times at various locations of pulmonary vessels, and sequence of X-ray planner projections are obtained. It is used to provide a definitive diagnosis when other imaging tests fail [4]. Although conventional pulmonary angiography has great value in PE diagnosis, it suffers from being expensive, invasive with serious side effect, requiring expertise and supporting staff, and not readily available in most hospitals.

Vascular Doppler ultrasound is a quick, noninvasive, and reliable technique [23]. It is painless and carries no risk. However, it provides less clinical information (e.g., number of clots and amount of obstruction) than other imaging techniques and very dependent on the experience of the examiner [4, 23].

Finally, several reports showed promising results for the assessment of PE with magnetic resonance imaging (MRI) [24, 25]. This modality is promising because images can be generated without radiation, and because it allows a combination of morphological and functional imaging (e.g., perfusion). However, MR has a lower spatial resolution than CT and much longer acquisition times (around 30 min as opposed to seconds in CT).

2.6. Treatment

Untreated PE can be fatal with high mortality rate that can be decreased under rapid detection [6]. There are ranges of different types of treatment procedures [4]. They include hemodynamic and respiratory support, anticoagulation medications, thrombolytic therapy, surgical embolectomy, percutaneous catheter-directed therapy, and venous filter intervention, which are not without complications. The selection of treatment depends on the PE severity and prognosis. Generally, the obstruction is mild when only a few subsegmental vessels are blocked and it is severe when multiple segmental or a few lobar vessels are blocked. Mild PE is managed with clot-dissolving medication. Severe PE requires additional medical intervention, such as placement of a filter in the inferior vena cava, or clot removal with either a catheter or surgery.

2.7. Summary

This section introduced clinical facts of pulmonary embolism. This includes concise of PE's epidemiology, predisposing factors, pathophysiology, classifications, and treatments procedures. The available diagnostic medical imaging systems, which are the decision-makers of the presence and severity of PE, were explained with their strengths and limitations, rationalizing the shift toward the use of CT.

3. Computerized tomography pulmonary angiography (CTPA)

Computerized tomography pulmonary angiography (CTPA) is a multidetector computerized tomography (MDCT) scanner that acquires cross-sectional chest images during the administration of contrast agent [10]. This permits the visualization of the blood flow in pulmonary veins and arteries. This section describes the CTPA technology and its impact in diagnosing PE. Aspects covered include: (1) the basic of CTPA technology, (2) the CTPA radiographic appearance, (3) the radiographic features of suspicious PE, and (4) the clinical performance of CTPA scans including sensitivity, specificity, and pitfalls.

3.1. CTPA technology

On CTPA, the patient's chest is exposed by a calibrated X-ray cone beam during the injection of contrast media into patient, as shown in **Figure 3**. The X-ray photons are absorbed (i.e., attenuated) by various structures within the chest. The amount of X-ray attenuations varies with accordance to the type and density of the tissues in the chest. The maximum absorption occurs in the dense bone and sites of contrast agent (i.e., pulmonary vessels); while the minimum absorption happens in the lung (i.e., air); the other thorax tissues (i.e., the heart, the muscles, and the upper parts of abdomen) lay in between those two structures. The X-ray

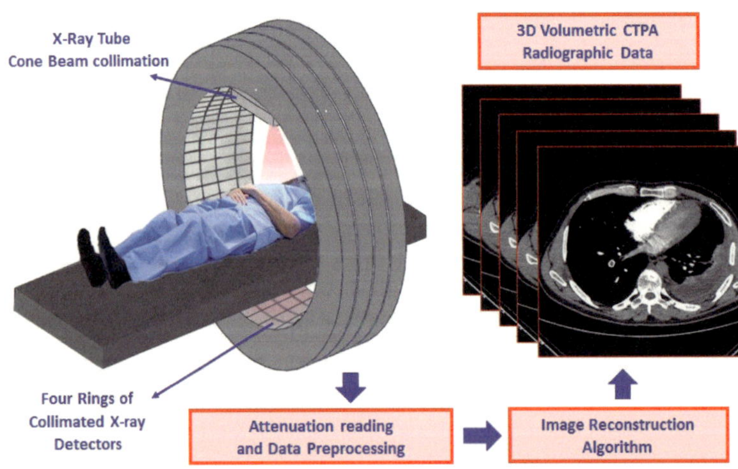

Figure 3. Four rings MDCT technology (there are 256 rings in modern MDCT).

cone beam rotates 360 degrees around the patient. At each angle, the penetrated X-ray beam from patient strikes rings of X-ray digital detectors. The detectors measure the amount of X-ray absorption and then fed to computer which, in turn, processes these data to reconstruct a CTPA three dimensional (3D) volumetric radiographic data of the chest's tissues. The CTPA image quality is governed by set of technical parameters; the interested readers may revise one of the MDCT books such as the book by Seeram in Ref. [26].

The volume of contrast media depends on patient weight, and may vary in [40 mL, 140 mL], also based on the dye concentration. Iodine is commonly used because of its relatively harmless interaction with the body and its solubility; the concentration is usually 250–350 mg/mL. Generally, a 4 or 5 mL/s is injected through a catheter in an antecubital vein. The rate of injection may increase in the advanced generations of MDCT, when acquisition time decreases in order to maintain sufficient iodine concentration within the vessels. The contrast peak happens after 10–25 s depending on the patient. Ideally, the scan should be complete before the radiographic dye reaches the left ventricle in the heart, as this may mean contrast has drained from the pulmonary arteries, or require a larger dose of contrast media.

3.2. CTPA radiographic appearance

The CTPA 3D radiographic data are displayed in three orthogonal views (i.e., Digital images); these are the two dimensional (2D) axial, sagittal, and coronal cross sections (**Figure 4**). In each CTPA view, the pixel brightness (2D picture element) is proportional to amount of X-ray absorption at tiny 3D cube (i.e., voxel) in the patient's chest.

Understanding the radiographic CTPA appearance is important during the detection of PE. The lung parenchyma exhibits the lowest X-ray absorption so it appears as "black" regions clearly delineating the borders of lungs in the CTPA view. The soft tissues (i.e., the heart, muscles, fat, and upper constituents of the abdomen) appear as a radiolucent area (lower X-ray absorption). These regions appear in a form of various radiographic shades of gray levels (i.e., various optical intensities). On contrast, the regions of bones and the contrast agent in the pulmonary vessels are radio-opaque (higher X-ray absorption) and appear as bright (i.e., white) regions. **Figure 4** demonstrates the radiographic appearance of these different tissues where the contrast agent (indicated by red letters "CA") looks brighter than the surrounding lung parenchyma, while remaining thorax constituents look with various intensities.

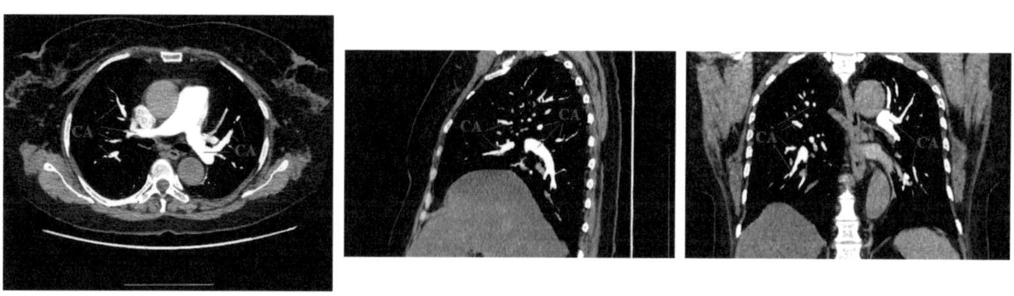

(a) (b) (c)

Figure 4. The three CTPA orthogonal views radiographic appearance (axial, sagittal, coronal).

3.3. PE radiographic features

The contrast medium opacifies the bloodstream in the lung. In case of PE, the pulmonary vessel is either completely blocked, or passes around it. Thus, on CTPA view, the veins and arteries appear white where the bloodstream is present, and a thrombus can be observed as a dark spot inside the white mass. **Figure 5** (left) illustrates examples of acute and chronic PE affecting the left main PA and right lobar artery, respectively. Acute thrombi appear as a hole, or concavity, in the vessel, while chronic clots are found on the edge of the vessel, with no concavity. **Figure 5** (right) also shows example of peripheral clot (segmental).

3.4. Clinical performance of CTPA scan

The radiologist navigates the CTPA slices searching the presence of a clot. The diagnosis of PE is categorized in a yes-or-no decision, independent of the location and severity of emboli. When a defect (clot) is found in one slice, the adjacent neighbors are analyzed. The radiologist tracks the clot to the point where she/he knows for sure its anatomical location in the pulmonary vascular veins and arteries and assesses his/her conclusion. Sensitivity and specificity are two statistical parameters commonly used to evaluate any diagnostic test. In this subsection, these two parameters are introduced in association with CTPA examination. This leads to the discussion of the CTPA artifacts.

3.4.1. Terminology background

Let us suppose that a population of patients, pathologically proved to have or not to have PE, was asked to undergo CTPA examination. Then, radiologists are asked to interpret these CTPA scans. The correct interpretation of a CTPA scan can be either a true-positive (TP) response (i.e., the correct detection of clots) or a true-negative (TN) response (i.e., the correct decision that there is no clot). In contrast, the false interpretation of a CTPA scan is described as either a false-positive (FP) response (i.e., the false suggestion of PE that does not exist) or a false-negative (FN) response (i.e., the PE is missed). These four possible categories of CTPA interpretation are illustrated in **Table 1**.

The proportion of TP responses to the total number of pathologically proven PE patients is referred as the true-positive fraction (TPF) or the sensitivity (the ability to detect patients with PE).

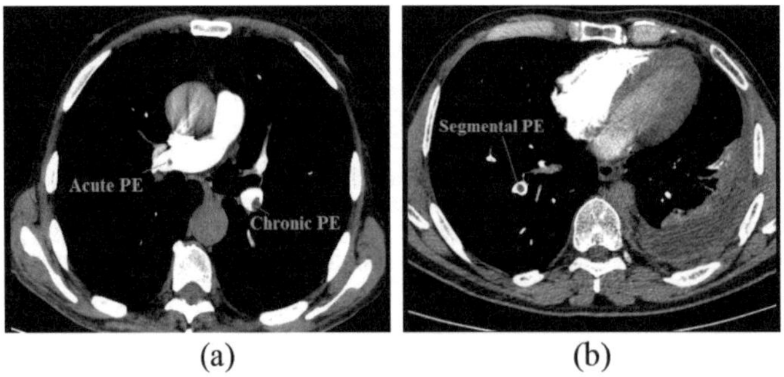

Figure 5. Examples of chronic and acute PE (left), and segmental PE (right) appearance on CTPA image.

	CTPA truth information	
Radiologist decision	**Abnormal (PE exists)**	**Normal**
Abnormal	True positive (TP)	False positive (FP)
Normal	False negative (FN)	True negative (TN)

Table 1. Outcomes of radiologist interpretation of CTPA examinations.

It is calculated as the ratio of TPs to the sum of FNs and TPs as illustrated in Eq. (1). On the other hand, the proportion of TN responses to the total number of patients, which do not have PE, is called the true-negative fraction (TNF) or specificity (the ability to exclude patients without PE). It is calculated as the ratio of TNs to the sum of FPs and TNs as illustrated in Eq. (2).

$$sensitivity = TPF = \frac{TP}{TP + FN} \tag{1}$$

$$specificity = \frac{TN}{TN + FP} \tag{2}$$

$$FPF = \frac{FP}{TN + FP} = 1 - specificity \tag{3}$$

Consequently, sensitivity measures the reader's performance in detecting patients with clots, whereas specificity measures the reader's ability to avoid producing false responses. Specificity is usually derived from the false-positive fraction (FPF) as shown in Eq. (3). Also, the predictive value of a positive test PV(+) and the predictive value of false test PV(−) can be evaluated as in Eqs. (4) and (5). These are also alternatively referred as positive predictive value (PPV) and negative predictive value (NPV). As FP and FN increase (i.e., increment in interpretation mistakes), the PPV and NPV decrease.

$$PV(+) = \frac{TP}{TP + FP} \tag{4}$$

$$PV(-) = \frac{TN}{TN + FN} \tag{5}$$

3.4.2. CTPA's sensitivity, specificity, and negative and positive predictive value

Early investigations were reported in the 1990s regarding the impact of CTPA examinations in detecting PE. The results of these reports were reviewed by Rathbun in 2000 [27] and Hiorns in 2002 [28], showing that the sensitivity and specificity of CTPA may vary between the range of 51–100 and 81–100%, respectively. These initial results revealed the possibility of MDCT to diagnose PE.

Over the last decade, the clinical role of CTPA examination has undergone extensive scientific investigations [7–10]. The largest and most significant collaborative clinical trial was conducted in 2006 [10]. This study is well-known as PIOPED II (Prospective investigation of pulmonary embolism diagnosis, second study). The dataset consisted of 824 patients who had enrolled for CTPA examination in the period 2001–2003 using 4, 8, and 16 rows MDCT devices. These CTPA scans were interpreted by different radiologists at remote clinical centers (i.e., hospitals) in the USA and Canada. The study reported sensitivity (i.e., the proportion of correct diagnosis of patients with PE) of 83% and specificity (i.e., the proportion of the correct diagnosis of patients without PE) of 96%. The high value of sensitivity means high TP and low FN (Eq. (1)), while high value of specificity means high TN and low FP (Eq. (2)). Based on the PE probability is low, intermediate, or high, the PPV and NPV was 58 and 96%, 92 and 89%, and 96 and 60%, respectively. On the other hand, based on the PE location is lobar, segmental, or subsegmental vessels, the PPV was 97, 68, and 25%, respectively. The defects at extreme sites of pulmonary vascular branches (segmental and subsegmental vessels) exhibit less observability, and consequently more challenging to radiologists, than lobar and main PA clots.

A recent report, in 2015, was published by Dogan et al. in the Netherlands; this study reviewed different CTPA clinical trials and reported that the sensitivity and specificity of CTPA scans may vary between the range of 83–100% and 89–96%, respectively [8]. The NPV was 96–99% showing the high CTPA scan's certainty in ruling out PE; *a negative CTPA can safely exclude PE*. Estrada-Y-Martin and Oldham supervised a survey regarding the clinical practice in the diagnosis of PE in USA [9]. The survey included members (i.e., Intervention Radiologists) of the Society of Thoracic Radiology (524 members) and the Society of Interventional Radiologists (389 members). The surveyed members believed that CTPA examination is the gold standard to diagnose PE. This conclusion sustained previous study emphasizing that CTPA is the first-line imaging for the evaluation of PE [7]. These clinical trials and surveys have resulted in the worldwide acceptance of CTPA as the best method for the detection of PE.

3.4.3. CTPA artifacts

Although the clinical reports accepted CTPA as best-reliable method with high sensitivity for diagnosing PE, their results also showed that FNs diagnosis, which are potentially life-threatening or a prospective health burden, may occur. For a radiologist, it can be difficult to detect all PE in the CTPA data [4, 10] for several reasons. In CTPA clinic, the radiologist is asked to examine stack of high resolution 2D CTPA images for single patient. Each 2D CTPA image is a 512 by 512 pixels. The stack builds a 3D CTPA volume of voxels (volume pixels), of which the size, in modern MDCT devices, is approximately 0.6 mm in every direction. Thus, a CTPA scan consists of millions of voxels have to be reviewed. Furthermore, the segmental and subsegmental vascular branches are quit complex; it is impossible to visualize all vascular structures within one CTPA image at a time. Therefore, radiologists usually revise the 3D CTPA volume several times examining only parts of the vascular system in the attempt not to miss an intravascular (sometimes very small) black dot indicating PE. A secure detection or exclusion of PE is therefore quite time-consuming and dependent on the experience of the radiologist.

Additionally, diagnostic pitfalls may occur due to CTPA artifacts [29, 30]. Some artifacts leads to defects that imitate PE; this may include a poorly filled vein with contrast media, lymphoid tissue around the vessels, impacted bronchi mimic dark tubular structures, or parenchymal diseases altering pulmonary perfusion. Technical factors may also lead to artifact hampering the correct PE diagnosis; this include image noise due to low dose or obese patients, respiratory or cardiac motion leading to inhomogeneous intravascular contrast, streak-artifacts near the superior vena cava due to beam hardening, incorrect timing resulting in insufficient intravascular contrast, or artifacts due to edge-enhancing image reconstruction. Further details of these artifacts are explained in MDCT technical books such as the reference number [26].

3.5. Summary

This section explained the CTPA practice. The CTPA basic physics, technology, examination, and radiographic appearance of PE and other thorax tissues were explained. The sensitivity, specificity, and PPV and NPV of CTPA are outlined based on clinical trials and surveys in the last two decades. These reports concluded that that CTPA remains, at the time, as the first line diagnostic procedure providing the less invasive procedure, and highest sensitivity, specificity, and NPV among other imaging techniques. The CTPA artifacts, which may contribute to misdiagnosis, were mentioned.

4. Computer-aided detection of PE on CTPA views

It is difficult and time consuming for a radiologist to navigate all CTPA orthogonal slices and find all emboli, this also depends on the radiologist experience. In PIOPED II, which was held at well-estimated clinical institutes, the average of 9.3% FP and 2.4 FN responses were reported [10]. This means that among 1000 suspicious PE patients, which is a daily small number of CTPA examination in any developed country, 93 patients may incorrectly diagnosed as having PE and may be asked to undergo further clinical tests, which is a clinical burden and probably additional X-ray radiation dose. Also, which is more critical, 24 patients may be incorrectly excluded of having PE and would leave the hospital without considering medication; these patients would be left under serious medical consequences that may be fatal. It is important to note again that FP and FN depend on radiologist experience, for example, in PIOPED II, it is possible for the NPV and PPV to be 58 and 60%, respectively. This lack of imperfection diagnosis may attribute to many reasons as explained in Section 3.4.3. Therefore, a computer-assisted detection (CAD) for the diagnosis of PE is desirable. This section aims to describe the CAD technology then explains the current state of how PE-CAD can contribute in improving patient health in CTPA clinic. This leads to explain the comments on CAD and the necessary recommendations. Comprehensive information on CAD technology in medical imaging can be found in Ref. [31].

4.1. CTPA-CAD definitions

A computer-aided detection (CAD) algorithm is an architecture of computer image analysis processes that yield, when applied to a CTPA examination, to the prompting of regions of suggestive pulmonary obstruction such as the presence of clots. Such prompting is often used as a "second opinion" to alert the radiologist to structures that, otherwise, might be overlooked [2, 3]. **Figure 6** shows a CTPA slice (left) and the responses of the CTPA-CAD (right), which are indicated as red overlay. They are also called as CAD stimuli, candidates, or outputs. These CTPA-CAD responses are categorized to one of four possible groups, similarly to those explained in Section 3.4.1 describing the radiologist accuracy in interpreting CTPA

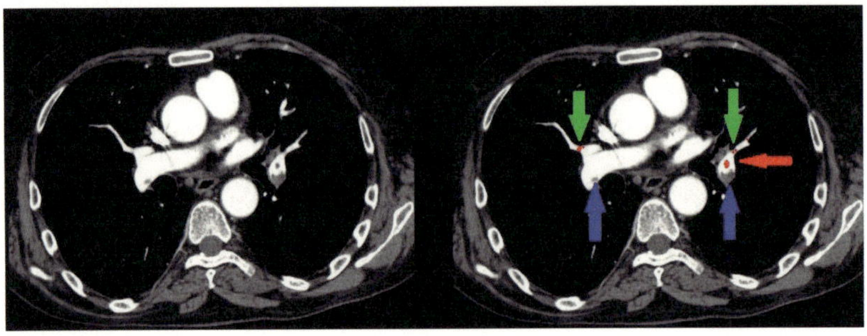

Figure 6. Types of assessment of CTPA-CAD stimuli on CTPA image.

scans. They are: the TP, FP, TN, FNs groups. **Figure 6** (right) illustrates TP (i.e., correct prompt of clot) and FP (incorrect prompt of clot) stimuli, indicated with red and green arrows, respectively. There are two clots that were not prompted, so they are FN stimuli, which are indicated with blue arrow. The remaining pulmonary vessels, which were not prompted as PE, are the TN stimuli. As with radiologist, it is desirable that a CTPA-CAD algorithm leads to the highest TP and TN, while it yields the lowest possible FP and FN stimuli.

The performance of the CAD software can be tested "per clot" or "per patient" basis. For "per clot" basis, the CTPA-CAD responses are counted in comparison to truth of all actual PE occurrences (i.e., all clots) in the CTPA examination. While for "per patient" basis, it is not important for the CTPA-CAD to find all thrombi. Additionally, the CTPA-CAD responses can be evaluated on "first reader" or "second reader" basis. The "first reader" analysis, which is also called as "standalone performance," refers to the outcomes of the CTPA-CAD software in a defined dataset of clinical CTPA scans *without* interference of radiologists. The "second reader" performance means that the CTPA-CAD output is utilized to support the radiologist decision *after* he/she has assessed the examination primarily unassisted and uses the results of CTPA-CAD only to refine his/her judgment.

As explained in Section 3.4, in current clinical CTPA practice, the diagnosis of PE is divided in a yes-or-no decision, regardless to the colts' number, location, and severity of emboli [4]. It is, therefore, less important that a CTPA-CAD system finds all emboli in a CTPA scan. More significant tasks of CTPA-CAD seem to be: to increase the radiologist's certainty to rule in or out PE (i.e., improve sensitivity and specificity), to reduce the CTPA interpretation time, and to decrease inter-reader variability [2, 3]. Thus, most researchers prefer the "per patient" basis to evaluate the performance of CTPA-CAD because it is more clinically relevant than the "per clot" basis.

4.2. CTPA-CAD performance

The first study on a CTPA-CAD algorithm was published in 2002 by Masutani et al. [32] for a group of 19 high-quality CTPA examinations; they reported a sensitivity on a *per clot* basis of 100% with 7.7 false-positive findings per examination. Since then, numerous methods, utilizing various image analysis concepts, have been tested by different vendors and image analysis groups. Some CTPA-CAD algorithms have attained clinical merit, while some are still under development. This section reviews the performance of these methods, dividing them into two groups. The first group describes the marketable CTPA-CAD available from famous vendors such as SIEMENS, PHILIPS, and GE. The second group describes underconstruction CTPA-CAD software. In general, the review focuses on the main image analysis aspects implemented in the CAD algorithm (if it was disclosed), the method's performance, size of dataset, and the characteristics of CTPA images, particularly the slice thickness that has direct impact on diagnosing PE.

4.2.1. *Commercial CTPA-CAD*

These are the CTPA-CAD methods that were developed at famous medical imaging vendors, for example, Philips (Philips Healthcare, Best, The Netherlands), Siemens (Siemens Medical Solutions, Germany), and GE (General Electric Healthcare, USA). They have been FDA approved and tested in a clinical environment. Since they are offered in the medical imaging market, the methodology (i.e., sequence of image analysis aspects) is not disclosed. This subsection presents the reports explaining their clinical performance "first reader" or "second reader" basis.

For CTPA-CAD made by *Philips*, two clinical trials by Wittenberg et al. [33, 34] and one by Lahiji et al. [35] were reported. The first trial by Wittenberg et al. was in 2010; they tested the CAD output on 225 negative and 67 positive CTPA scans (292 retrospective scans) acquired from 16 and 64 MDCT devices with 0.9 or 1 mm slice thickness [33]. For "first reader" basis, the results showed 94 and 21% sensitivity and specificity, in turn. The rate of FP stimuli was 4.7 per examination. The NPV was 92% indicating possibility to serve as reassurance for less experienced readers. The CAD also found seven FN scans, two at segmental and five at subsegmental vessels. The second trial was published in 2012 [34]. They examined the performance of six radiologists with and without the CTPA-CAD on 158 negative and 51 positive retrospective CTPA scans, which were obtained from 16 and 64 MDCT devices with 0.9 or 1 mm slice thickness. For "second reader" basis, there was no significant change in specificity, but the sensitivity increased in the range from 12% (expert reader) to 12 (radiologist-in-training or less expert). The rate of FP was 4.9 per scan. Lahiji et al., in 2014 [35], evaluated 26 negative and 40 positive CTPA scans from 256 MDCT device with 0.9 mm slice thickness. Although their study was to compare two different CTPA image reconstruction algorithms (the iterative and filtered back projection techniques), a CTPA-CAD software was used for the assessment. For "first reader" basis, the reported sensitivity and specificity for both image reconstruction techniques were in the range 85–97.2 and 26.9–61.5, respectively. The rate of FP was in the range 1.5–3.6.

For CTPA-CAD made by *Siemens*, Lee et al. studied 16 negative and 21 positive CTPA scans acquired from dual energy CT angiography (DCTA) with 1.2 mm slice thickness [36]. When both readers used the CAD prototype, the sensitivity was improved by approximately of 5% without significant loss in specificity. The rate of FP was 3.5 per examination. Blockmon et al. evaluated 79 CTPA scans (36 positive and 43 negative) from 16 and 64 CTPA devices at 1 mm slice thickness [37]. The radiologists, without the aid of CTPA-CAD, scored 84.4 and 92.6 sensitivity and specificity, in turn. For "first reader" basis, the CTPA-CAD achieved 93.8% sensitivity and 14.9% specificity; while it achieved 92.2% and 88.3% for "second reader" basis. The FP rate was 3.5 per scan. Earlier study was by Engelke et al. in 2008 [38]. They studied 56 positive CTPA scans obtained from 64 MDCT device with 0.6-mm slice thickness. On "second reader" basis, the four readers reported no significant loss of specificity while sensitivity increased in the range 3–7%. The FP rate was 4.1 per scan.

Wittenberg et al. compared the performance of three different CTPA-CAD systems made by *Philips, GE,* and *Siemens* [39]. They studied three groups of CTPA scans from 64 MDCT devices made in Philips, GE, and Siemens with 0.6, 0.9, and 1.5 mm slice thickness, in order. The three groups of dataset contained 38, 39, and 38 positive CTPA scans; it also contained 40, 40, 37 negative CTPA scans, respectively, according to each CTPA group. For "first reader" basis, the comparison yielded a sensitivity of 100, 97, and 92, specificity of 18, 15, and 13, and FP rate of 4.5, 6.2, and 3.7, respectively, to each group.

Table 2 summarizes the results of previous trials of different CTPA-CAD systems from different vendors. For comparison, the table also includes the results from PIOPED II (the largest clinical trial) explained in Section 3.4.2. The table illustrates the CTPA clinical performance once CTPA images are interpreted by the radiologist, the CTPA-CAD software (CAD first Reader basis), consensus between radiologist and the CTPA-CAD software (CAD second reader basis). The table consists of 7 main columns. The first column shows the author with the reference number. The second column indicates the interpretation procedure type (radiologist, the CTPA-CAD software, consensus of Radiologist and the CTPA-CAD software). The third column demonstrates the dataset's size indicating the number of positive and negative CTPA scans. The fourth, fifth, and sixth column indicate the performance in term of sensitivity, specificity and rate of FP, in order. Finally, the last column shows slice thickness used to acquire CTPA image. **Table 3** shows the range values of the sensitivity, specificity, and FP rate for each diagnosis protocol, which are reported in **Table 2**.

The findings listed in **Tables 2** and **3** indicate the following:

1. If CTPA scan is interpreted by radiologist only, the sensitivity and specificity may not reach 100%. The sensitivity range from 77.7% (for radiologist-in-training or less experience) to 94% (expert radiologist). While the specificity varies in the range 89–98% indicating almost perfect performance in excluding PE. The 100% specificity reported by Lee et al. [36] (**Table 2**) was reported on small number of negative CTPA scans, so it cannot be generalized.

2. For CTPA-CAD "first reader" basis, the marketable CTPA-CAD methods can score reliable high sensitivity, which can exceed the performance of an expert radiologist. However, the specificity is low (~20% in all reports in **Table 2**) due to 3.4–4.9 FP stimuli per CTPA scan. The 61.5 specificity reported by Lahiji et al. [35] is concluded from applying iterative reconstruction that is under research.

3. For CTPA-CAD "second reader" basis, the CAD can improve radiologists' sensitivity up to 7%. This increment in sensitivity coincides with no significant change in specificity. This enhancement can be substantial for inexperienced radiologist as reported by Wittenberg et al. [34], which one of the radiologists scored 90% with the aid of CTPA-CAD in comparison to 78% without the CAD assistance.

4. The results were obtained on different MDCT devices, thus the performance of CTPA-CAD is independent of scanner type. However, it is relevant to image quality and scanning protocols such as slice thickness. Actually, the slice thickness has significant impact on PE diagnosis. For example, Jung et al. [40] analyzed 15 positive and 25 negative CTPA scans acquired with slice thicknesses of 0.625, 1.3, and 2.5 mm from 64 MDCT device. As

Author	CTPA interpretation protocol	Dataset size		Sensitivity (%)	Specificity (%)	FP rate per scan	Slice thickness (mm), MDCT device
		Positive CTPA	Negative CTPA				
PIOPED II [10]	Radiologists	192	632	83	96	Not applicable	1.25 4, 8, 16 rows MDCT
Wittenberg [34]		51	158	78–94	89–98		0.9–1.0 16, 64 rows MDCT
Lee [36]		21	16	90.9	93.3–100		1.2 DCTA
Blackmoon [37]		36	43	84.4	92.6		1.0 16, 64 rows MDCT
Engelke [38]		56	—	77–93	—		0.6 64 rows MDCT
Wittenberg [33]	CTPA-CAD *Philips*, Siemens, or GE	67	225	94	21	4.7	0.9–1.0 16, 64 rows MDCT
Lahiji [35]		40	26	85–97.5	26.9–61.5	1.5–3.6	0.9 256 rows MDCT
Blackmoon [37]		36	43	93.8	14.9	3.5	1.0 16, 64 rows MDCT
Wittenberg [39]		38	40	100	18	4.5	0.6 64 rows MDCT
Wittenberg [39]		39	40	97	15	6.2	0.9 64 rows MDCT
Wittenberg [39]		38	37	92	13	3.7	1.5 64 rows MDCT
Wittenberg [34]	Consensus between Radiologist and CTPA-CAD	51	158	90–96	91–98	4.9	0.9–1 16, 64 MDCT
Lee [36]		21	16	95.5	93.3–100	3.5	1.2 DCTA
Blackmoon [37]		36	43	92.2	88.3	3.5	1.0 16, 64 rows MDCT
Engelke [38]		56	—	84–96	—	4.1	0.6 64 rows MDCT

Table 2. "Per patient" CTPA interpretation by the radiologist, "first reader" marketable CTPA-CAD software, and "second reader" CTPA-CAD software, showing sensitivity, specificity, rate of FP responses, and the characteristics of dataset used in the clinical trials.

CTPA interpretation protocol	Sensitivity (%)	Specificity (%)	FP rate per scan
Radiologists	77–94	89–98	—
CAD (Philips, Siemens, or GE)	85–100	13–61.5	1.5–6.2
Consensus between radiologist and CAD (Philips, Siemens, GE)	84–96	88.3–100	3.5–4.9

Table 3. "Per patient" range of the values of sensitivity, specificity, rate of FP responses, based on each protocol of CTPA interpretation.

slice thickness increases, there was significant decrease of PE diagnosis of lobar, segmental, subsegmental clots on both the axial and coronal CTPA views. They concluded that a slice thickness of 1 mm is a must to achieve high sensitivity, particularly the subsegmental PE. This impact is applicable to CTPA-CAD and must be considered in any CAD prototype [2, 3]. This matter, among other variables, is further described in Section 4.3.

Consequently, the marketable CTPA-CAD software can increase reader sensitivity for the detection of PE, particularly the segmental and subsegmental pulmonary clots, and enforce reader confidence for the diagnosis of PE without significant loss of specificity. This rise in sensitivity means less FN CTPA scans (Eq. (1)), thus improving patient health.

4.2.2. Underconstruction CTPA-CAD

There are nonmarketable CAD systems under construction by researchers. They share the employment of CTPA pulmonary vessels segmentation, candidate clot detection, and texture and feature computation with/without morphology analysis on 2D and 3D levels. However, they explored recent advances in computer sciences to reduce the FP rate such as complex mathematical classifier [41–43] and artificial intelligence (e.g., neural networks) [44, 45]. Thus, they reported their results on "per clot" basis.

The results in **Table 4** demonstrate that the "per clot" CTPA-CAD's sensitivity is in the range from 63–80%. This qualifies those CAD prototypes to be tested on "per patient" basis. However, the rate of FP stimuli is still high, so a low specificity value, as those in **Table 2**, is again very likely to happen. False-positive stimuli are the main burden hindering radiologist from accepting the

Author	Number of clots in CTPA cases	Sensitivity (%)	FP rate per scan
Bouma [41]	318 in 57 positive CTPA	63	4.9
Zhou [42]	595 in 59 positive CTPA	80	22.6
Zhou [43]	537 in 50 positive CTPA (PIOPED II)	80	8.6
Park [44]	44 in 18 positive CTPA	63.2	18.4
Tajbakhsh [45]	326 in 121 positive CTPA	83	2

Table 4. "Per clot" sensitivity and FP rate for underconstruction CTPA-CAD prototypes.

superfluous sensitivity of CTPA-CAD. To reduce the FP rate, Tajbakhsh [45] employed 3D presentation of PE and blood vessels, coupled to neural network, to produce 2 FP per CTPA scan (**Table 4**). Al-hinnawi et al. [46] suggested another 3D technique, but simpler than neural networks that requires training and calibration on dataset characteristics, to reduce the FP rate. In the final step of their CTPA-CAD system, the stimuli from three CTPA views were orthogonally recombined to produce a single *interactive 3D display of PE candidates* from the CTPA case, as illustrated in **Figure 7**. Thus, this would permit, in a single analysis instead of slice by slice analysis, the assessment of CAD performance on the aggregated CAD responses on the three CTPA views of each patient. This could reduce time, and consequently reduce burden to radiologist. Clots that are bigger in size than 1 mm^3 were retained based on the voxel size of the CTPA scan. Thus, the CAD system can be tuned in accordance with the variations in CTPA acquisition settings due to patient differences, which was not employed in previous marketable CTPA-CAD systems or underconstruction CTPA-CAD prototypes. This reduces the variations in CAD outputs due to variation in patient preparation such as slice thickness. They reported that this approach would reduce the FP rate of from CAD systems, such as those in **Tables 2** and **4**, by 30% while it increases or ascertains the correct rate of CTPA-CAD's TP stimuli as much as 27%.

4.3. Factors affecting CTPA-CAD performance

CTPA-CAD systems are image quality dependent [2, 3, 47, 48]. As for any X-ray imaging technique, the CTPA image quality is ruled by factors related to subject variance, acquisition parameters, patient preparation, and dose management [4, 49]. The subject variances such as

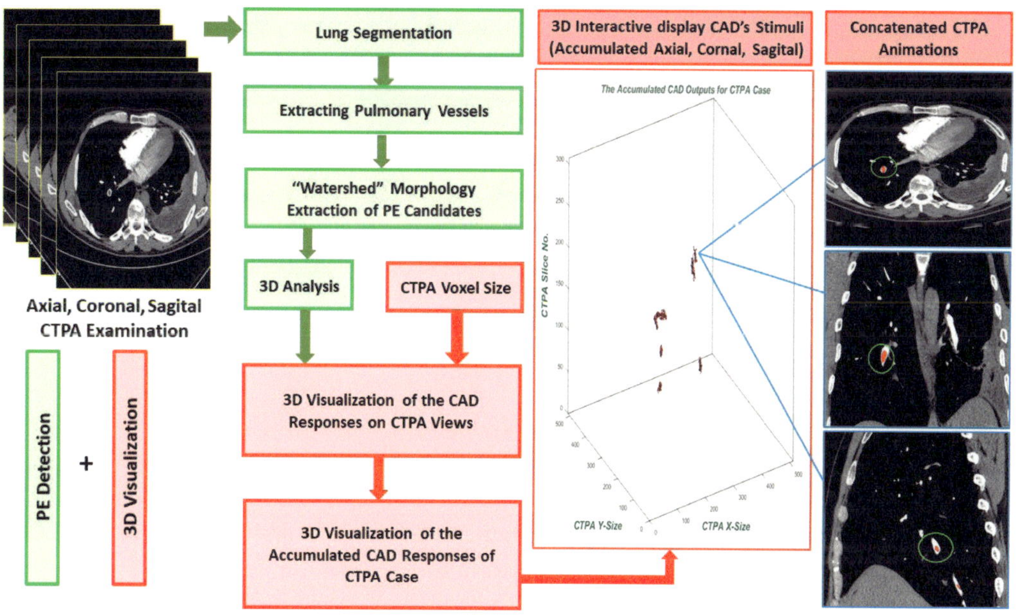

Figure 7. Three dimensional visualization of CTPA-CAD output (courtesy from radiological physics and technology no. JSMP30–180024).

age, sex, race, presence of risk factors, prevalence and morphology of the clots, they do *not* have impact on CTPA image quality; so they should not influence the CTPA-CAD outcome. Thus, there is no need to calibrate the CAD system based on different patients or countries.

However, the acquisition and patient preparation variables are fundamental factors in CTPA image quality. They may lead to bias in the CTPA-CAD output [2, 3, 47–49]. Acquisition parameters include KV, mA, type of reconstruction algorithm, accurate MDCT window, and any post processing filtration, among other technical parameters, they all affect CTPA image contrast. On the other hand, patient preparation include mainly the slice thickness, correct contrast agent dose and rate of injection, and accurate timing to acquire CTPA images during the pulmonary vessels are filled with contrast agent not after it drained to heart, they all affect the precise depiction of clots with variable sizes and locations [4, 7, 10, 40]. While radiologist, and the clinical physicist or radiographer, may be relatively unaware to such factors, it is believed for sure that they have direct impact on CAD systems because they lead to alterations in the representation of radiographic features on which CAD relies [2, 3, 48, 50].

Dose management also has crucial role on any CAD output. As reducing X-ray dose is main concern in imaging, different vendors provide imaging protocols and reconstruction techniques to reduce patient dose without substantially risking the image quality. These ultra-low dose, or even low dose, settings lead to lower contrast to noise ratio, which in turn leads to higher possibility to CT artifacts and lower capability to spot diseases [51–53]. These parameters are relevant to any CAD system [2, 3, 47, 48], so can greatly affect the PE CAD performance.

4.4. CTPA-CAD recommendations

Therefore, subsequently to the discussion mentioned earlier, the CTPA-CAD manufactures should clearly describe the operating characteristics of their PE CAD prototypes. This include, the supported range of equipment, CTPA image acquisition settings, patient preparation requirements, reconstruction algorithms, and patient special cases such as those with additional lung defects, among other relevant factors, that radiologist need to be aware during the use of CTPA-CAD. Additionally, in case of CTPA-CAD comparison with findings from previous CTPA scans is used to assess decisions on diagnosis, disease progression, and/or treatment effectiveness, care must be considered to match the acquisition conditions accordingly to CTPA-CAD operating manual [2, 3, 47–53].

4.5. Summary

This section described the current status of utilizing PE CAD prototypes in CTPA clinic. The necessity of CAD systems in PE diagnosis is highlighted, and different possible CAD group of outputs are explained. Then, according to research centers from different countries, the performance of marketable and underdevelopment CTPA-CAD systems is elucidated. The PE CAD performance can be described according to "per clot" or "per patient" basis, and "first reader" or "second reader" basis. The "per patient" basis is more relevant to CTPA clinical practice than "per clot". Both the "first reader" and "second reader" basis lead to high sensitivity that can reach 100%, outweighing the radiologist performance. However, the specificity drops dramatically and become much less than the radiologist performance in case of "first reader" basis. Studies showed that the best operating scenario is the "second reader" basis because it improves sensitivity, which means less FN results, while it guarantees no significant change in specificity, in comparison to human observer performance. The factors affecting the CTPA-CAD output were described at the end of this section, this yielded to suggest recommendation.

5. Conclusion

This chapter presents comprehensive *current status* knowledge in the PE angiography clinic. The clinical proofs of thrombosis are explained in Section 2. Knowledge of PE epidemiology, predisposing factors, pathophysiology, classifications, diagnostic medical imaging modalities, and treatments procedures are described. Then, in Section 3, concentration is focused on describing the CTPA technology that is the clinically accepted as the best first-line imaging procedure in PE diagnosis because it is fast, lowest invasive, and the highest sensitivity procedure, among other medical imaging modalities. Issues covered are CTPA physics, technology, examination, radiographic appearance, and PE features, the clinical trials in term of sensitivity, specificity, PPV, and NPV, are explained. Section 4 provides demonstration of the art of CAD system and their influence on improving the PE diagnoses by being eligible to reduce miss diagnosis by radiologist. Advantages and disadvantages of assessing CTPA-CAD performance with regard to "per patient", "per clot", "first reader", and "second reader" basis are explained. Results suggested that the "second reader" along with "per patient" basis is the best scenario to utilize PE CAD systems, because this raises the sensitivity without effect on specificity of radiologist performance. Precautions and recommendations of optimal practice of PE CAD prototypes are described indicating the necessity to follow the operation manual specifications, particularly the CTPA acquisition parameters and patient preparation, which the CAD relies on.

Acknowledgements

Thanks with appreciation are due to Mrs. Haneen Kharayseh and Ms. Ayah Bittar, Architecture Engineering Department at the Hashemite University, for their cooperation in the production of **Figures 1–3**.

Author details

Abdel-Razzak M. Al-hinnawi

Address all correspondence to: hinawiabed@hu.edu.jo

Faculty of Allied Health Sciences, Medical Imaging Department, The Hashemite University, Zarqa, Jordan

References

[1] Litjens G, Kooi T, Babak Bejnordi E, Setio AA, Ciompi F, Ghafoorian M, van der Laak JAWM, Ginneken B, Sánchez CI. A survey on deep learning in medical image analysis. Medical Image Analysis. 2017;**42**:60-88

[2] Petrick N, Sahiner B, Armato SG, Bert A, Correale L, Delsanto S, Freedman MT, Fryd D, Gur D, Huo Z, Jiang Y, Morra L, Paquerault S, Raykar V, Samuelson F, Summers RM, Tourassi G, Yoshida H, Zheng B, Zhou C, Chan HP. Evaluation of computer-aided detection and diagnosis systems. Medical Physics. 2013;**40**(8):087001

[3] Tang J, Agaian S, Thompson I. Guest editorial: Computer-aided detection or diagnosis (CAD) systems. IEEE Systems Journal. 2014;**8**(3):907-908

[4] Konstantinides SV, Torbicki A, Agnelli G, Danchin N, Fitzmaurice D, Galie N, Gibbs JSR, Huisman MV, Humbert M, Kucher N, Lang I, Lankeit M, Lekakis J, Maack C, Mayer E, Meneveau N, Perrier A, Pruszczyk P, Rasmussen LH, Schindler TH, Svitil P, Noordegraaf AV, Zamorano JL, Zompatori M. 2014 ESC guidelines on the diagnosis and management of acute pulmonary embolism. European Heart Journal. 2014;**35**:3033-3069

[5] Heit JA. The epidemiology of venous thromboembolism in the community. Arteriosclerosis, Thrombosis, and Vascular Biology. 2008;**28**:370-372

[6] Mathers CD, Loncar D. Projections of global mortality and burden of disease from 2002 to 2030. PLoS Medicine. 2006;**3**(11:e442):2011-2030. DOI: 10.1371/journal.pmed.0030442

[7] Cronin P, Weg JG, Kazerooni EA. The role of multidetector computed tomography angiography for the diagnosis of pulmonary embolism. Seminars in Nuclear Medicine. 2008;**38**:418-431

[8] Dogan H, de-Roos A, Geleijins J, Huisman MV, Kroft LJM. The role of computed tomography in the diagnosis of acute and chronic pulmonary embolism. Diagnostic and Interventional Radiology. 2015;**21**:307-316

[9] Estrada-Y-Martin RM, Oldham SA. CTPA as the gold standard for the diagnosis of pulmonary embolism. International Journal of Computer Assisted Radiology and Surgery 2011;**6**:557-563

[10] Stein PD, Fowler SE, Goodman LR, Gottschalk A, Hales CA, Hull RD, Leeper KV, Popovich J, Quinn DA, Sos TA, Sostman HD, Tapson VF, Wakefield TW, Weg GJ, Woodard PK. Multidetector computed tomography for acute pulmonary embolism. The New England Journal of Medicine. 2006;**354**(22):2317-2327

[11] Wells PS, Ginsberg GS, Anderson DR, Kearon C, Gent M, Turpie AG, Bormanis J, Weitz J, Chamberlain M, Bowie D, Barnes D, Hirsh J. Use of a clinical model for safe management of patients with suspected pulmonary embolism. Annals of Internal Medicine. 1998;**129**(12):997-1005

[12] Goldhaber SZ, Morrison RB. Pulmonary embolism and deep vein thrombosis. Circulation, American Heart Association. 2002;**106**(12):1436-1438

[13] Temgoua1 MN, Tochie JN, Noubiap JJ, Agbor VN, Danwang C, Endomba1 FTA, Nkemngu NJ. Global incidence and case fatality rate of pulmonary embolism following major surgery: A protocol for a systematic review and meta-analysis of cohort studies. Systematic Reviews. 2017;**6**:240-245. DOI: 10.1186/s13643-017-0647-8

[14] Akgüllü C, Ömürlü IK, Eryılmaz U, Avcil M, Dağtekin E, Akdeniz M, Güngör H, Zencir C. Predictors of early death in patients with acute pulmonary embolism. The American Journal of Emergency Medicine. 2015;**33**:214-221

[15] Raskob GE, Angchaisuksiri P, Blanco AN, Buller H, Gallus A, Hunt BJ, Hylek EM, Kakkar A, Konstantinides SV, McCumber M, Ozaki Y, Wendelboe A, Weitz JI, ISTH Steering Committee for World Thrombosis Day. Thrombosis: A major contributor to global disease burden. Arteriosclerosis, Thrombosis, and Vascular Biology. 2014;**34**(11):2363-2371. DOI: 10.1161/atvbaha.114.304488. PMID 25304324

[16] Rahimtoola A, Bergin JD. Acute pulmonary embolism: An update on diagnosis and management. Current Problems in Cardiology. 2005;**30**(2):61-114. DOI: 10.1016/j.cpcardiol.2004.06.001. PMID 15650680

[17] Kosacka U, Kiluk IE, Milewski R, Tycińska AM, Jasiewicz M, Sobkowicz B. Variation in the incidence of pulmonary embolism and related mortality depending on the season and day of the week. Polskie Archiwum Medycyny Wewnętrznej. 2015;**125**:92-94

[18] Vazquez FJ, Posadas-Martinez ML, Vicens J, Bernaldo de Quiros FG, Giunta DG. Incidence rate of symptomatic venous thromboembolic disease in patients from a medical care program in Buenos Aires, Argentina: A prospective cohort. Thrombosis Journal. 2013;**11**:16

[19] Ghaye B, Ghuysen A, Bruyere PJ, D'Orio V, Dondelinger RF. Can CT pulmonary angiography allow assessment of severity and prognosis in patients presenting with pulmonary embolism? What the radiologist needs to know. Radiographics. 2006;**26**:23-39

[20] Ghaye B, Ghuysen A, Willems V, Lambermont B, Gerard P, D'Orio V, Gevenois PA, Dondelinger RF. Severe pulmonary embolism: Pulmonary artery clot load scores and cardiovascular parameters as predictors of mortality. Radiology. 2006;**239**(3):884-891

[21] Sinzinger H, Rodrigues M, Kummer F. Ventilation/perfusion lung scintigraphy. Multiple applications besides pulmonary embolism. Hellenic Journal of Nuclear Medicine. 2013;(1):50-55

[22] Nguyen NC, Abdelmalik A, Moinuddin A, Osman MM. Detection of pulmonary embolism: Comparison of methods. Journal of Nuclear Medicine. 2010;**51**(5):823-824

[23] Zanobetti M, Bigiarini S, Coppa A, Conti A, Innocenti F, Pini R. Usefulness of chest ultrasonography in detecting pulmonary embolism in patient with chronic obstructive pulmonary disease and chronic renal failure: A case report. The American Journal of Emergency Medicine. 2012;**30**:1665.e1-1665.e3. DOI: 10.1016/j.ajem.2011.09.021

[24] Hosch W, Schlieter M, Ley S, Heye T, Kauczor HU, Libicher M. Detection of acute pulmonary embolism: Feasibility of diagnostic accuracy of MRI using a stepwise protocol. Emergency Radiology. 2014;**21**:151-158. DOI: 10.1007/s10140-013-1176-y

[25] Bannas P, Bell LC, Johnson KM, Schiebler ML, François CJ, Motosugi U, Consigny D, Reeder SB, Nagle SK. Pulmonary embolism detection with three-dimensional Ultrashort Echo time MR imaging: Experimental study in canines. Radiology. 2016;**278**(2):413-421

[26] Seeram E. Computed Tomography: Physical Principle, Clinical Applications, Quality Control. 3rd ed. Missouri, USA: Elsevier; 2009. ISBN: 978-1-4160-2895-6

[27] Rathbun SW, Raskob GE, Whitsett TL. Sensitivity and specificity of helical computed tomography in the diagnosis of pulmonary embolism: A systematic review. Annals of Internal Medicine. 2000;**132**:227-232

[28] Hiorns MP, Mayo JR. Spiral computed tomography for acute pulmonary embolism. Canadian Association of Radiologists Journal. 2002;**53**(5):258-268

[29] Karabulut N, Kıroğlu Y. Relationship of parenchymal and pleural abnormalities with acute pulmonary embolism: CT findings in patients with and without embolism. Diagnostic and Interventional Radiology. 2008;**14**:189-196

[30] Wittram C, Maher MM, Yoo AJ, Kalra MK, Shepard JO, McLoud TC. MDCT angiography of pulmonary embolism: Diagnostic criteria and causes of Misdiagnosis1. Radiographics. 2004;**24**:1219-1238

[31] Li Q, Nishikawa RM. Computer-Aided Detection and Diagnosis in Medical Imaging. Boca Raton, FL, USA: CRC Press; 2015. ISBN 9781439871768

[32] Masutani Y, MacMahon H, Doi K. Computerized detection of pulmonary embolism in spiral CT angiography based on volumetric image analysis. IEEE Transactions on Medical Imaging. 2002;**21**(12):1517-1523

[33] Wittenberg R, Peters JF, Sonnemans JJ, Prokop M, Schaefer-Prokop CM. Computer-assisted detection of pulmonary embolism: Evaluation of pulmonary CT angiograms performed in anon-call setting. European Radiology. 2010;**20**:801-806

[34] Wittenberg R, Berger FH, Peters JF, Weber M, Hoorn F, Beenen LFM, Doorn M, Schuppen J, Zijlstra IJ, Prokop M, Schaefer-Prokop CM. Acute pulmonary embolism: Effect of a computer assisted detection prototype on diagnosis-an observer study. Radiology. 2012;**262**(1):305-313 [132]

[35] Lahiji K, Kligerman S, Jeudy J, White C. Improved accuracy of pulmonary embolism computer-aided detection using iterative reconstruction compared with filtered back projection. AJR. 2014;**03**:763-771

[36] Lee CW, Seo JB, Song JW, Kim MY, Lee HY, Park YS, Chae EJ, Jang YM, Kim N, Krauss B. Evaluation of computer-aided detection and dual energy software in detection of peripheral pulmonary embolism on dual-energy pulmonary CT angiography. European Radiology. 2011;**21**:54-62

[37] Blackmon KN, Florin C, Bogoni L, McCain JW, Koonce JD, Lee H, Bastarrika G, Thilo C, Costello P, Salganicoff M, Schoepf UJ. Computer-aided detection of pulmonary embolism at CT pulmonary angiography: Can it improve performance of inexperienced readers? European Radiology. 2011;**21**:1214-1223

[38] Engelke C, Schmidt S, Bakai A, Auer F, Marten K. Computerassisted detection of pulmonary embolism: Performance evaluation in consensus with experienced and inexperienced chest radiologists. European Radiology. 2008;**18**:298-307

[39] Wittenberg R, Peters JF, Weber M, Cobben LP, Prokop M, Schaefer-Prokop CM. Standalone performance of a computer assisted detection prototype for detection of acute pulmonary: A multi-institutional comparison. The British Journal of Radiology. 2012;**85**:758-764

[40] Juang IJ, Kim KJ, Ahn MI, Kim HR, Park HJ, Jung SH, Lim HW, Park SH. Detection of pulmonary embolism using 64-slice multidetector row computed tomography: Accuracy and reproducibility on different image reconstruction parameters. Acta Radiologica. 2011;**52**:417-421

[41] Bouma H, Sonnemans JJ, Vilanova A, Gerritsen FA. Automatic detection of pulmonary embolism in CTA images. IEEE Transactions on Medical Imaging. 2009;**28**(8):12231230

[42] Zhou C, Chan HP, Sahiner B, Hadjiiski LM, Chughtai A, Patel S, Wei J, Cascade PN, Kazerooni EA. Computer-aided detection of pulmonary embolism in computed tomographic pulmonary angiography (CTPA): Performance evaluation with independent data sets. Medical Physics. 2009;**36**(8):3385-3394

[43] Zhou C, Chan HP, Chughtai A, Kuriakose JW, Kazerooni EA, Hadjiiski LM, Wei J, Patel S. Robustness evaluation of a computer-aided detection system for pulmonary embolism (PE) in CTPA using independent test set from multiple institutions. In: Hadjiiski LM, Tourassi GD, ed. Medical Imaging. Computer-Aided Diagnosis. Proc. of SPIE Vol. 941408-1. https://doi.org/10.1117/12.2082015

[44] Park SC, Chapman BE, Zheng B. A multistage approach to improve performance of computer-aided detection of pulmonary embolisms depicted on CT images: Preliminary investigation. IEEE Transactions on Biomedical Engineering. 2011;**58**(6):1519-1527

[45] Tajbakhsh N, Gotway MB, Liang J. Computer-aided pulmonary embolism detection using a novel vessel-aligned multiplanar image representation and convolutional neural networks. In: Medical image computing and computer-assisted intervention MICCAI 18th International Conference, Munich, Germany, October 5-9, 2015, Proceedings, Part II 9350. pp. 62-69. https://doi.org/10.1007/978-3-319-24571-3_8

[46] Al-hinnawi AR, Al-Naami BO, Al-azzam H. Collaboration between interactive three-dimensional visualization and computer aided detection of pulmonary embolism on computed tomography pulmonary angiography views. Radiological Physics and Technology. 2018;**11**:61-72

[47] Doi K. Computer-aided diagnosis in medical imaging: Historical review, current status and future potential. Computerized Medical Imaging and Graphics. 2007;**31**:198-211

[48] Nishikawa RM, Pesce LL. Computer-aided detection evaluation methods are not created Equal1Radiology. Radiology. 2009;**251**(3):634-636

[49] Lee CS, Nagy PG, Weaver SJ, Newman-Toker DE. Cognitive and system factors contributing to diagnostic errors in radiology. AJR. 2013;**201**:611-617

[50] Huo Z, Summers RM, Paquerault S, Lo J, Hoffmeister J, Armato SG III, Freedman MT, Lin J, Lo SCB, Petrick N, Sahiner B, Fry D, Yoshida H, Chan HP. Quality assurance and training procedures for computer-aided detection and diagnosis systems in clinical use. Medical Physics. 2013;(40):1-13

[51] Lee ES, Kim SH, Im JP, Kim SG, Shin C, Han JK, Choi BI. Effect of different reconstruction algorithms on computer-aided diagnosis (CAD) performance in ultra-low dose CT colonography. European Journal of Radiology. 2015;**84**:547-554

[52] Lo P, Young S, Kim HJ, Brown MS, McNitt-Gray MF. Variability in CT lung-nodule quantification: Effects of dose reduction and reconstruction methods on density and texture based features. Medical Physics. 2016;**43**(8):4854-4865

[53] Yanagawa M, Honda O, Kikuyama A, Gyobu T, Sumikawa H, Koyama M, Tomiyama N. Pulmonary nodules: Effect of adaptive statistical iterative reconstruction (ASIR) technique on performance of a computer-aided detection (CAD) system—Comparison of performance between different-dose CT scans. European Journal of Radiology. 2012;**81**:2877-2886